USE IT OR LOSE IT

Ultimate face yoga guide

BINDU GARG

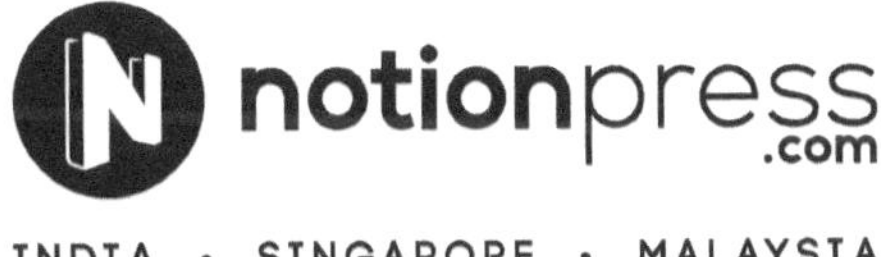

INDIA • SINGAPORE • MALAYSIA

ACKNOWLEDGMENTS

I extend my heartfelt gratitude to my husband, Varun Garg, for his unwavering support, patience, and belief in me at every step of this journey. A special thank you to my wonderful mother, whose endless motivation and encouragement have been my greatest inspiration. My deepest love and appreciation go to my kids for their constant love and joy, which fuel my determination.

My sincere appreciation goes to The Shubh Yoga Foundation for providing invaluable testimonies and unwavering support that helped shape this work.

To my family and friends – your kindness, motivation and belief in me have been a true blessing. This journey would not have been the same without each of you. Thank you for being part of it and making this milestone so special.

A heartfelt tribute to my beloved father, whose blessings have guided me every step of the way. Had he been here today, I know he would have been immensely proud of this achievement, and his joy would have made this milestone even more special.

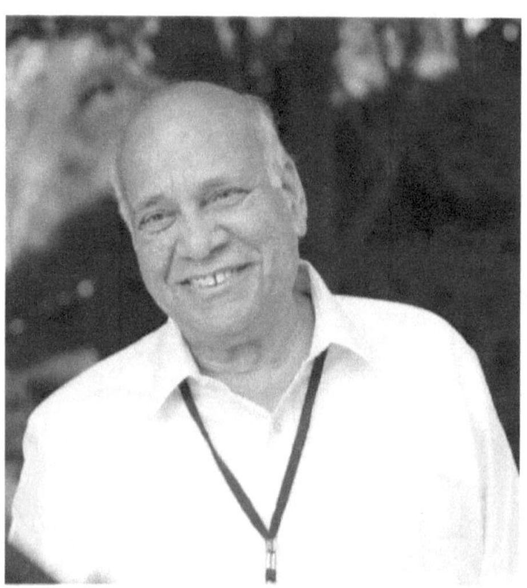

CONTENTS

◁ Contents ▷

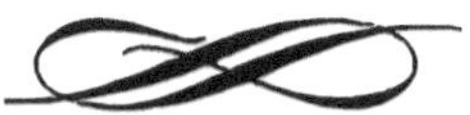

FOREWORD

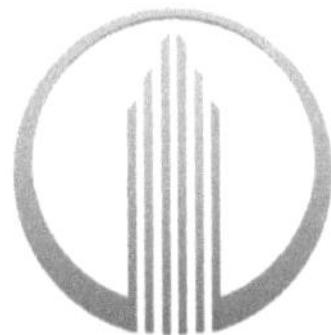

It is a privilege to write this foreword for "Use It or Lose It: The Ultimate Face Yoga Guide", authored by the remarkably insightful Bindu Garg. This book is not just a guide—it's a revelation. It speaks directly to our times, when people are seeking ways to reclaim their health, beauty, and balance naturally, without invasive methods or superficial fixes.

Bindu Garg presents face yoga not just as a series of exercises, but as a powerful tool for self-awareness, healing, and inner alignment. Her approach is thoughtful, practical, and rooted in authentic experience. She has taken something ancient and spiritual and made it accessible, engaging, and deeply relevant to every reader—regardless of age or background.

What strikes me most is her sincerity. This book comes not from theory, but from passion, practice, and personal conviction.

I congratulate Bindu Garg for this meaningful and timely contribution. May her work inspire thousands to rediscover their natural vitality and confidence—one breath, one pose, one moment at a time.

– Rakesh Goyal
Chairman
Real Estate Regulatory Authority (RERA)

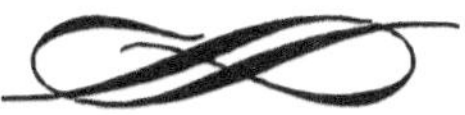

INTRODUCTION TO FACE SCULPTING WITH FACE YOGA

Just like the muscles in your body, your facial muscles need regular movement and exercise to stay firm and toned. If you neglect them, they weaken over time, leading to sagging skin, wrinkles, and loss of definition—hence the phrase "Use it or lose it."

A well-defined, sculpted face is often associated with youth, vitality, and confidence. While many people turn to skincare products, cosmetic procedures, and invasive treatments to achieve these results, an ancient yet highly effective method is gaining renewed recognition—Face Yoga. This holistic approach to facial sculpting harnesses the power of targeted exercises, massage techniques, and mindful movements to tone, lift, and rejuvenate the face naturally.

The Art and Science of Face Sculpting

Face Yoga is based on the principle that the muscles in our face, just like those in our body, require exercise to stay firm and toned. With over 40 muscles in the face and neck, these areas can be trained to maintain elasticity, improve circulation, and reduce sagging. By engaging in a consistent practice, one can achieve a naturally sculpted, youthful appearance without relying on invasive procedures.

Scientific research supports the idea that facial exercises can enhance muscle strength, improve skin elasticity, and increase collagen production. A 2018 study published in JAMA Dermatology found that participants who practiced facial exercises regularly for 20 weeks experienced improved facial fullness and a more youthful appearance. This growing body of evidence highlights the effectiveness of Face Yoga as a powerful, non-invasive alternative to modern anti-aging treatments.

Why Face Yoga?

Face Yoga is not just about aesthetics; it is a holistic wellness practice that combines mindfulness, breathwork, and self-care. Here are some of its key benefits:

- Natural Face Sculpting: Strengthens and tones facial muscles, enhancing definition in areas like the jawline, cheekbones, and eyes.
- Improved Skin Health: Boosts blood circulation, promoting a healthy glow and better nutrient delivery to the skin.
- Reduced Signs of Aging: Helps smooth wrinkles, fine lines, and sagging by stimulating collagen and elastin production.
- Relaxation and Stress Reduction: Relieves tension stored in the facial muscles, which can contribute to wrinkles and dull skin.
- Non-Invasive & Cost-Effective: Offers a natural, safe alternative to cosmetic procedures with long-term results when practiced consistently.

What to Expect in This Book

This book is designed to be a comprehensive guide to face sculpting with Face Yoga, covering everything from foundational techniques to advanced exercises for targeted concerns. Whether you are looking to achieve a more lifted look, reduce puffiness, or enhance your natural beauty, this guide will provide you with:

- Understanding Facial Anatomy: Learn how the muscles of the face work and why they play a crucial role in sculpting.
- Step-by-Step Face Yoga Exercises: Detailed instructions on how to perform each exercise correctly.
- Massage and Lymphatic Drainage Techniques: Reduce bloating, detoxify the skin, and improve facial contours.
- Breathwork and Mindfulness Practices: Enhance the effectiveness of Face Yoga by integrating relaxation techniques.
- Skincare Tips: Support your Face Yoga practice with holistic beauty and wellness advice.

By the end of this book, you will have all the knowledge and tools needed to incorporate Face Yoga into your daily routine and achieve a naturally sculpted, youthful face.

Let's embark on this journey of self-care, empowerment, and transformation—one facial movement at a time.

UNDERSTANDING FACIAL ANATOMY FOR FACE SCULPTING

To sculpt and tone the face effectively using Face Yoga, it is essential to understand the anatomy of the face—how its muscles, skin, and underlying structures work together to shape our appearance. Unlike the muscles in the body, which are anchored to bones at both ends, facial muscles are unique because they are attached to the skin. This allows them to control facial expressions, movement, and the overall structure of the face.

By gaining insight into facial anatomy, you can target specific muscles to lift, tone, and sculpt different areas of your face naturally. This chapter will provide an in-depth look at the key components of the face, including muscles, skin, fat pads, bones, and connective tissues, all of which influence your facial structure and appearance.

1. The Muscles of the Face: The Foundation of Sculpting

The human face contains over 40 muscles, each playing a vital role in expressions, movement, and support. These muscles can be strengthened and toned, just like those in the body, to create a more sculpted appearance.

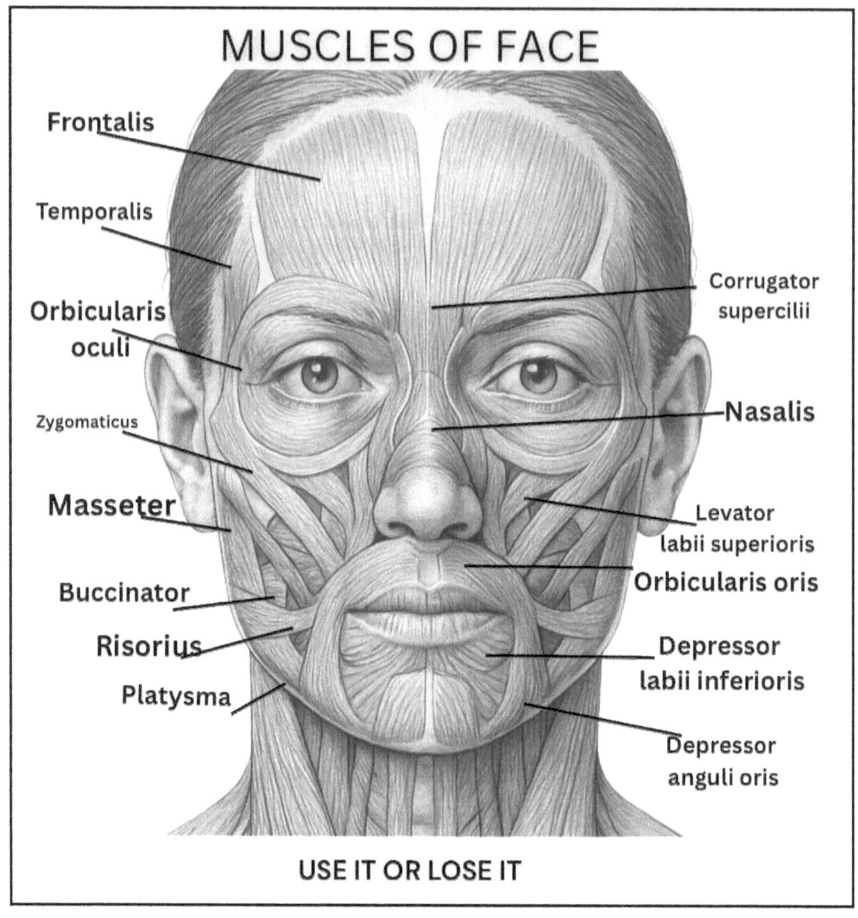

Key Facial Muscle Groups

1. Forehead & Eye Area

- Frontalis: Runs across the forehead and is responsible for raising the eyebrows and creating forehead lines.
- Orbicularis Oculi: A circular muscle around the eyes that controls blinking, squinting, and closing the eyelids. Strengthening it can help reduce drooping and fine lines.
- Corrugator Supercilii: Located between the eyebrows, this muscle is responsible for frown lines (the "11" wrinkles).

2. Cheeks & Mid-Face

- Zygomaticus Major & Minor: These muscles lift the corners of the mouth, contributing to smiling and cheek contouring.
- Buccinator: Found in the cheeks, this muscle controls movements like puffing and sucking and helps maintain facial volume.
- Levator Labii Superioris: Helps in lifting the upper lip, contributing to a youthful smile.

3. Mouth & Jawline

- Orbicularis Oris: A circular muscle around the lips that controls movements like puckering, kissing, and speaking.
- Depressor Anguli Oris: Pulls the corners of the mouth downward, contributing to a "sad" expression when overactive.
- Masseter: One of the strongest muscles, located at the jaw, which plays a role in chewing and jaw tension.
- Platysma: A sheet-like muscle extending from the jawline down the neck, essential for tightening the neck and preventing sagging.

How Face Yoga Strengthens Facial Muscles

Just as weight training helps tone body muscles, Face Yoga exercises engage and activate facial muscles, preventing atrophy, sagging, and wrinkles. By consistently working these muscles, you can redefine your facial contours and improve overall symmetry.

2. The Skin: Layers & Elasticity

The skin is the largest organ of the body and serves as the outermost layer of the face. It plays a significant role in appearance, as healthy, firm skin enhances the results of Face Yoga.

Layers of the Skin

- Epidermis: The outermost layer that protects the skin from environmental damage and contains melanin, responsible for skin tone.
- Dermis: The middle layer, rich in collagen and elastin, which gives the skin firmness and flexibility.
- Hypodermis (Subcutaneous Tissue): The deepest layer containing fat cells that provide cushioning and shape.

How Face Yoga Benefits the Skin

- Boosts blood circulation, improving skin nourishment and creating a natural glow.
- Stimulates collagen and elastin production, helping to reduce wrinkles and sagging.
- Encourages lymphatic drainage, eliminating toxins and reducing puffiness.

3. The Role of Fat Pads in Facial Structure

The fat pads in the face contribute to facial volume and shape. As we age, these fat pads shift or decrease, leading to hollowness, sagging, and loss of definition.

Main Facial Fat Pads

- Malar Fat Pad (Cheek Area): Gives the cheeks a youthful, plump appearance.
- Buccal Fat Pad (Mid-Cheek): Provides volume to the lower cheeks and jawline.
- Submental Fat (Under Chin): Accumulation in this area can lead to a double chin, which Face Yoga can help tone.

Face Yoga helps by strengthening muscles underneath the fat pads, providing natural lift and reducing sagging.

4. The Facial Bone Structure: The Framework

Beneath the muscles, skin, and fat pads, the facial bones form the fundamental structure of the face. The size and shape of the bones influence facial contours, including the jawline, cheekbones, and forehead.

Key Facial Bones for Sculpting

- Zygomatic Bone (Cheekbone): Defines the cheek area.
- Mandible (Jawbone): Determines the sharpness of the jawline.
- Maxilla (Upper Jaw): Supports the mid-face structure.

How Face Yoga Supports Bone Health

- Increases bone density by stimulating circulation around the bones.
- Strengthens the muscle attachments, improving facial definition.

5. Connective Tissue & Fascia: The Hidden Sculpting Factor

The fascia is a thin layer of connective tissue that lies between the muscles and skin, holding everything in place. When fascia becomes tight due to stress, poor posture, or aging, it can cause facial sagging and stiffness.

Face Yoga & Fascia Release

Face Yoga, combined with facial massage techniques, releases tension in the fascia, improving flexibility, circulation, and overall facial tone.

Conclusion: The Foundation for Face Sculpting

Understanding facial anatomy is the first step in mastering Face Yoga for natural face sculpting. By targeting specific muscles, improving skin elasticity, preserving fat distribution, supporting bone structure, and enhancing fascia health, Face Yoga provides a holistic and scientific approach to achieving a lifted, youthful, and sculpted face.

In the next chapters, we will explore specific Face Yoga exercises that engage these facial components, helping you achieve a naturally contoured and radiant look—without invasive treatments.

FACIAL EXERCISES

Forehead Exercises

The frontalis muscle is a broad, thin muscle located in the forehead. It plays a crucial role in lifting the eyebrows and creating forehead expressions, such as surprise or worry. However, repeated movement of the frontalis muscle can lead to horizontal forehead lines and premature wrinkles. By performing targeted Face Yoga exercises, you can tone, strengthen, and smooth this muscle, reducing wrinkles and lifting the brows naturally.

Why Strengthen the Frontalis?

- Lifts sagging eyebrows and prevents droopy eyelids
- Reduces forehead wrinkles and fine lines
- Improves blood circulation, enhancing skin elasticity
- Prevents tension headaches caused by forehead strain

1. The Forehead Smoother

This exercise trains the frontalis to move without creating deep horizontal lines, preventing premature aging.

How to Perform:

1. Apply light facial oil or serum.
2. Apply gentle pressure and slowly sweep your hands outward toward the temples.

3. While doing this, try not to raise your eyebrows—instead, focus on relaxing the forehead.
4. Repeat 10 times, breathing deeply.

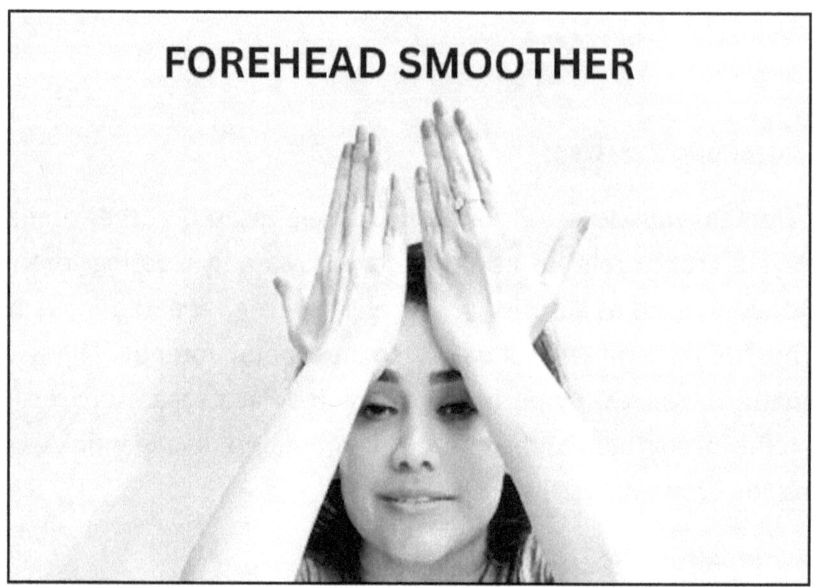

Benefits:

- Relaxes overactive forehead muscles
- Smooths existing forehead lines
- Enhances blood circulation for youthful skin

2. The Resistance Lift

This exercise tones the frontalis muscle while preventing sagging of the brows and eyelids.

How to Perform:

1. Place both index fingers above your eyebrows.
2. Gently press down to create resistance.

3. Try to lift your eyebrows upward against the pressure.
4. Hold for 5 seconds, then relax.
5. Repeat 10 times.

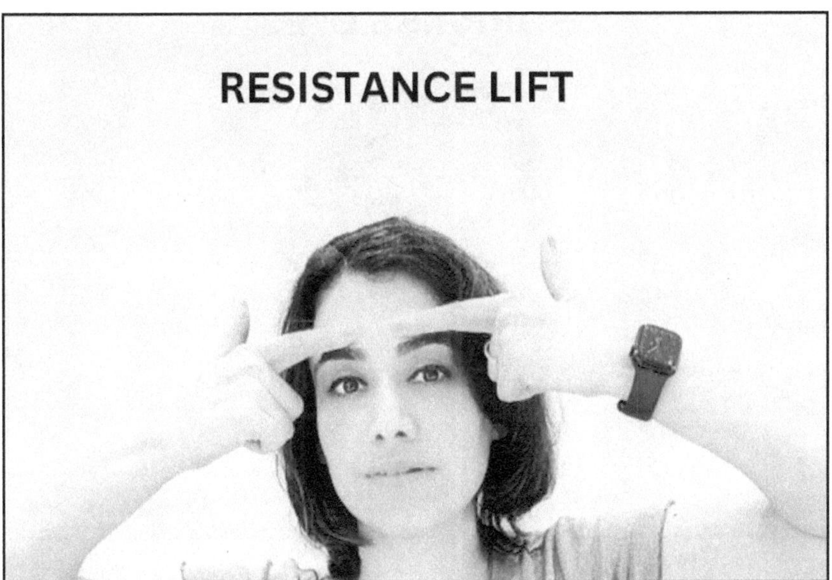

Benefits:

- Strengthens the frontalis without overuse
- Lifts drooping eyebrows and eyelids
- Trains the muscle to function correctly without excessive movement

3. Surprise Eyes

This exercise helps tone the forehead without creating horizontal lines.

How to Perform:

1. Open your eyes as wide as possible, like you're surprised.
2. Keep your forehead smooth—do not raise your eyebrows.

3. Hold the position for 10 seconds, then relax.
4. Repeat 5-7 times.

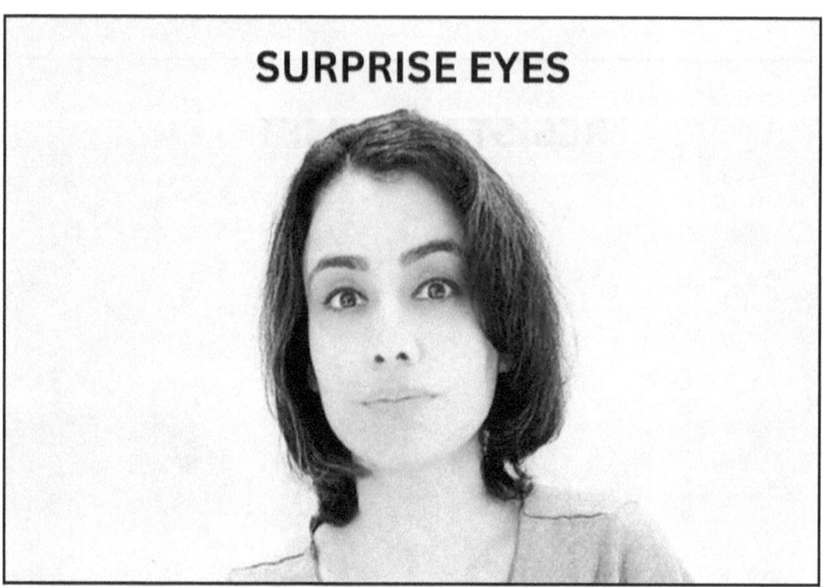

Benefits:

- Strengthens the forehead without creating wrinkles
- Trains the muscles to open the eyes without excessive brow lifting
- Reduces forehead tension and improves elasticity

4. Forehead Rub Face

How to Perform:

1. Place both palms or fingertips on your forehead.
2. Your fingers should rest horizontally across the forehead, just above your eyebrows.
3. Apply Gentle Pressure
4. Press your fingers or palms lightly onto your forehead.

5. Avoid pressing too hard; keep the movement gentle and soothing
6. Move from the center of your forehead outward toward the temples.
7. Repeat this for 30-60 seconds in a continuous motion.

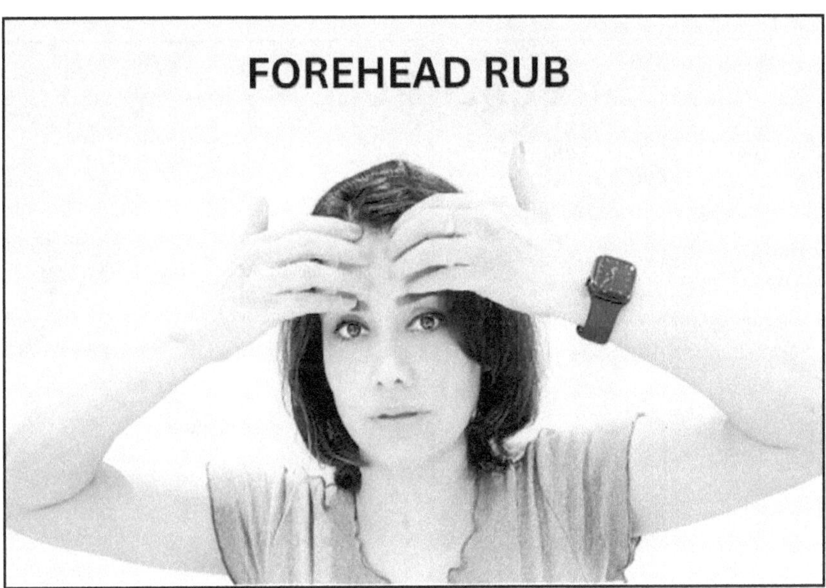

Benefits:

- Reduces forehead lines and wrinkles
- Relaxes forehead muscles, preventing expression lines
- Boosts blood circulation, promoting a healthy glow
- Relieves tension headaches and stress
- Promotes lymphatic drainage, reducing puffiness

5. The Scalp Pull (For a Lifted Forehead & Hairline)

This technique activates the frontalis and improves circulation to the scalp, promoting a youthful forehead and even healthy hair growth.

How to Perform:

1. Place your fingertips at the front of your scalp near the hairline.
2. Gently pull the scalp back and hold for 5 seconds.
3. Release and repeat 10 times.

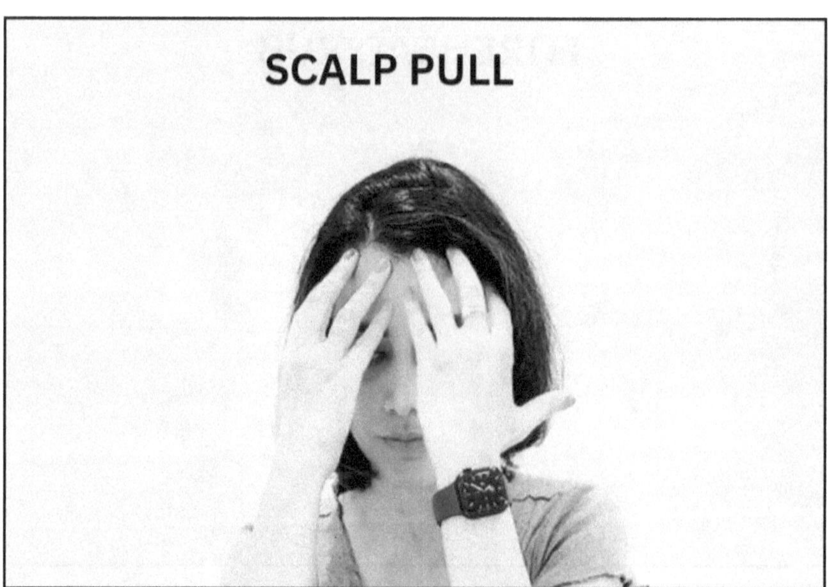

Benefits:

*   Lifts the forehead naturally
*   Improves circulation to the scalp and skin
*   Prevents sagging of the forehead over time

6. Zigzag

How to Perform:

1. Place the index and finger of both hands on the centre of your forehead. Your fingers should rest horizontally, just above the eyebrows.

2. Press lightly but firmly on the skin. Keep your forehead relaxed—avoid raising your eyebrows. Create the Zigzag Motion

3. Move your fingers in a zigzag pattern across the forehead.

4. Start from the centre and move outward toward the temples.

5. Ensure the movement is gentle yet firm, without stretching the skin.

6. Repeat the Motion. Perform this zigzag movement 5-10 times across the forehead. Take slow, deep breaths as you massage.

7. After the zigzag motion, use both palms to gently glide upward from the eyebrows to the hairline.

8. This ensures a lifting and relaxing effect on the frontalis muscle.

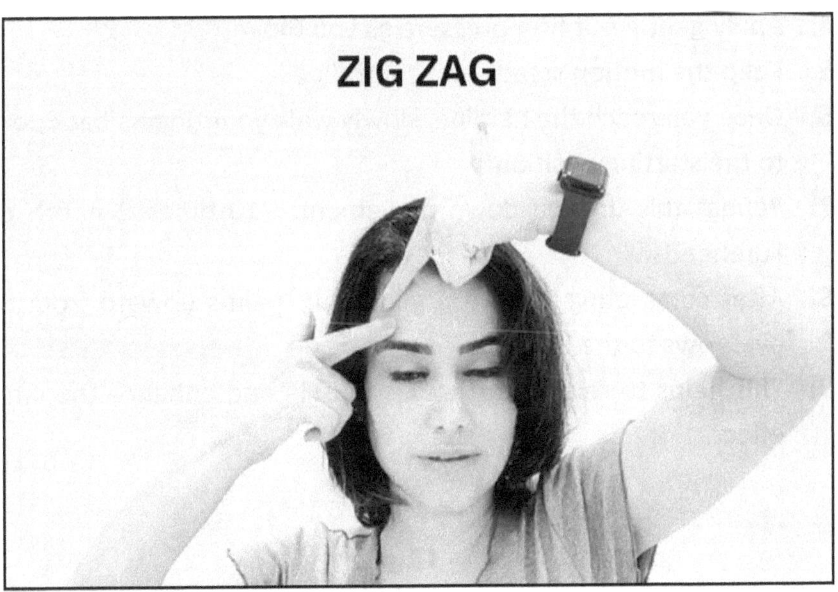

Benefits:

- Tones and strengthens the frontalis muscle
- Reduces horizontal forehead lines and wrinkles
- Releases tension and stress, preventing expression lines

- Boosts circulation, promoting a fresh, youthful glow
- Encourages lymphatic drainage, reducing puffiness

7. Forehead Walk

How to Perform:

1. Place the index, little and middle fingers of both hands on the forehead, just above the eyebrows.
2. Keep your hands lightly pressed against the skin without pulling.
3. Using your fingers, walk them slowly upwards toward the hairline in small steps.
4. Apply gentle but firm pressure as you move.
5. Keep the motion steady and controlled.
6. Once you reach the hairline, slowly walk your fingers back down to the starting position.
7. Repeat this up and down movement 5-10 times. Smooth the Forehead
8. After completing the walk, glide your palms upward from the eyebrows to the hairline.
9. This helps to relax the frontalis muscle and enhance the lifting effect.

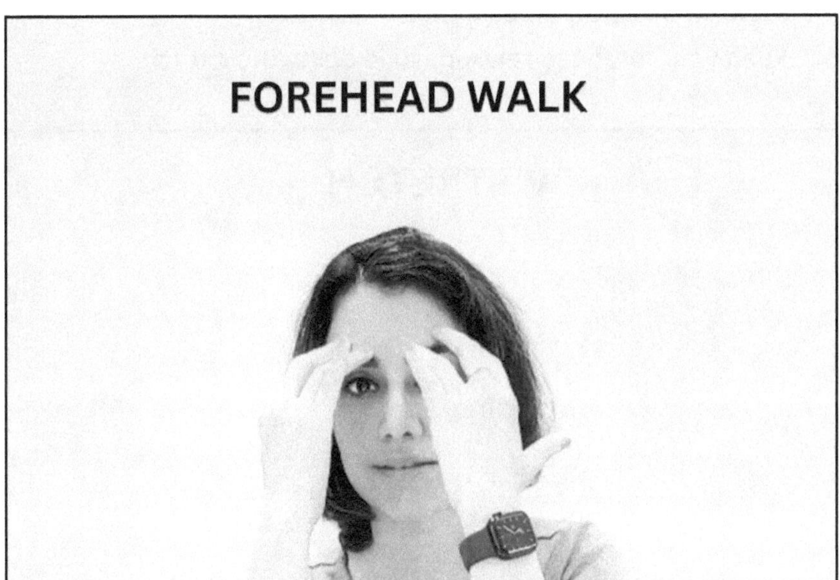

Benefits:

- Strengthens the frontalis muscle for a toned forehead
- Reduces horizontal forehead wrinkles and fine lines
- Encourages blood circulation, giving a natural glow
- Releases stress and tension, preventing expression lines
- Lifts and firms the forehead, improving skin elasticity

8. V-Stretch

How to Perform:

1. Place your index and middle fingers in a "V" shape at the center of your eyebrows.
2. Gently press and glide the fingers outward toward the temples.
3. Feel a mild stretch across the forehead, but avoid pulling too hard.

4. Perform this 5-10 times for best results.
5. Keep your forehead relaxed while doing the stretch.

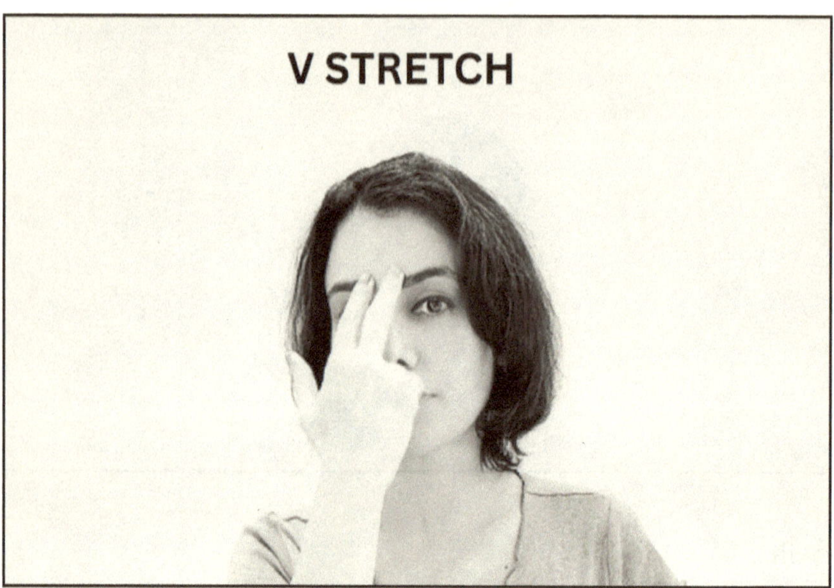

Benefits:

- Reduces frown lines and forehead wrinkles
- Opens up the eye area, making eyes appear brighter
- Improves blood circulation, promoting skin rejuvenation
- Releases tension from the forehead and eye region

9. Forehead line eraser

The Forehead Line Eraser Exercise is a powerful technique to smooth forehead wrinkles by lifting, stimulating circulation, and draining excess fluid. Here's how to do it effectively:

How to Perform:

1. Apply a light facial oil or serum to allow smooth gliding.
2. Sit comfortably with a relaxed posture.
3. Pinch, Use your thumb and index fingers of both hands to gently pinch the skin just above your eyebrows.
4. Lift the skin slightly to release tension from the forehead muscles.
5. Glide Towards the Temples. Maintain a light but firm pressure to encourage lymphatic drainage.
6. Repeat, Continue pinching and gliding across the entire forehead, working from the centre outwards.
7. Perform this motion 5–10 times for optimal results.
8. Once done, gently press and hold your fingers on the temples for a few seconds to aid relaxation and drainage.

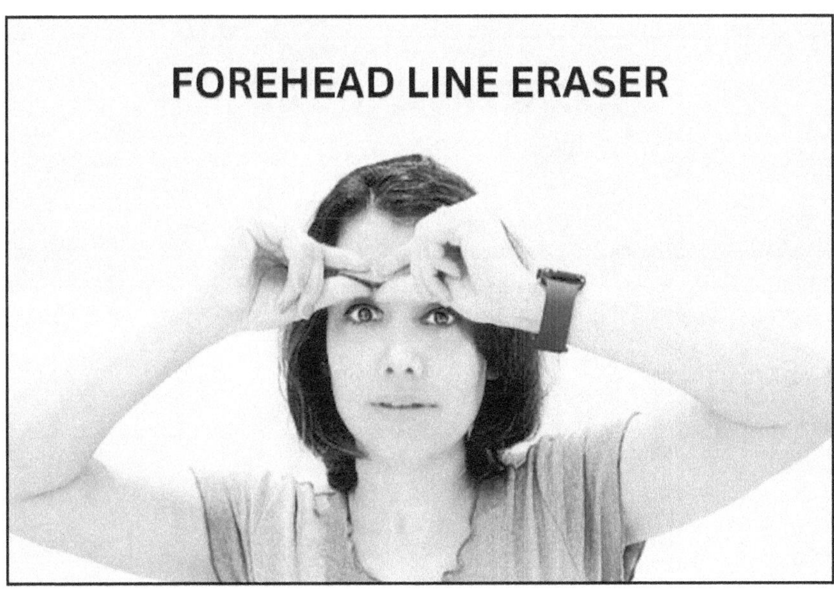

Benefits:

- Smooths fine lines and wrinkles

- Relieves forehead tension
- Stimulates circulation and collagen production
- Enhances lymphatic drainage to reduce puffiness

10. Forehead Hold

How to Perform:

1. Place both palms firmly on your forehead, covering the entire area.
2. Try to lift your eyebrows while using your hands to resist the movement.
3. Hold for 10–15 seconds, feeling the tension in your forehead muscles.
4. Release and relax for a few seconds.

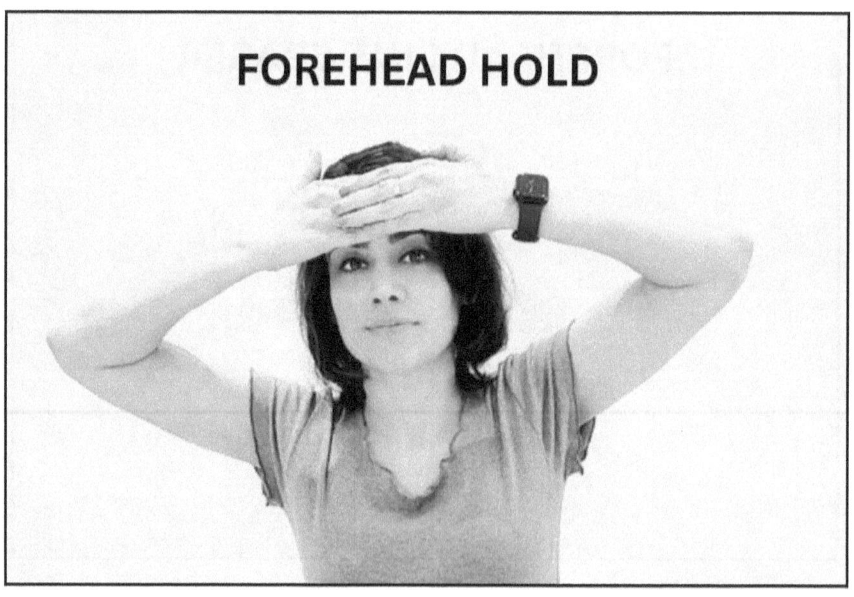

Benefits: Strengthens the forehead muscles while preventing excessive creasing.

11. Forehead Massage & Lymphatic Drainage (Releases Tension & Enhances Skin Glow)

When massaging the forehead for lymphatic drainage and sculpting, the key is to use gentle, rhythmic strokes to encourage fluid movement while also relaxing tension. Here are some effective strokes:

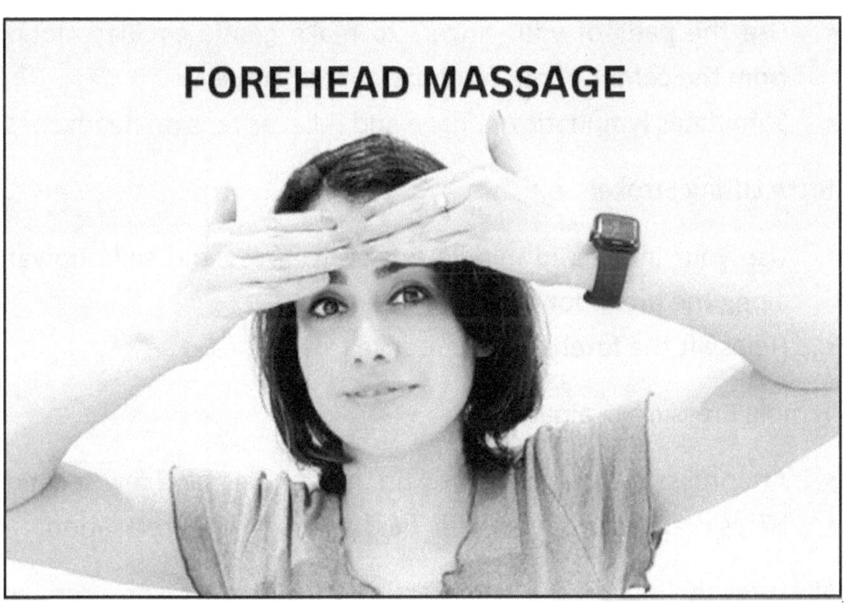

1. Upward Lifting Strokes

- Use your fingertips or knuckles to gently glide upward from the eyebrows to the hairline.
- Helps smooth forehead lines and promotes circulation.

2. Sweeping Drainage Strokes

- Place your fingers in the center of your forehead and sweep outwards towards the temples.
- Enhances lymphatic flow and reduces puffiness.

3. Zigzag Knuckle Massage

- Use the knuckles or fingertips to make small zigzag movements across the forehead.
- Relieves muscle tension and softens fine lines.

4. Circular Lymphatic Strokes

- Use the pads of your fingers to make gentle circular motions from the center of the forehead to the temples.
- Stimulates lymphatic drainage and relieves tension headaches.

5. Brow Lifting Stroke

- Use your index and middle fingers to press and slide upwards along the brow bone.
- Helps lift the forehead and reduce frown lines.

6. Temple Pressure Drainage

- After massaging, press gently on the temples for a few seconds.
- Helps drain excess lymphatic fluid and promotes relaxation.

For best results, always use light pressure with a facial oil or serum, and repeat each stroke about 5–10 times.

Conclusion

The frontalis muscle plays a vital role in facial expressions, eyebrow positioning, and forehead movement. By incorporating targeted Face Yoga exercises, you can:

- Strengthen & tone the forehead for a naturally lifted appearance.
- Prevent and reduce forehead wrinkles by training the muscle to function correctly.
- Enhance circulation & relaxation, promoting smoother, younger-looking skin.

With consistent practice, these Face Yoga techniques can help you maintain a firm, youthful, and wrinkle-free forehead—naturally!

In the next chapter, we will explore Face Yoga exercises for the eye area, helping to reduce crow's feet, under-eye puffiness, and droopy eyelids. Let's continue sculpting a youthful, radiant face—one exercise at a time!

Eye Exercises

The orbicularis oculi is a circular muscle surrounding the eyes, responsible for blinking, squinting, and closing the eyelids. Over time, aging, stress, and repetitive movements lead to crow's feet, under-eye bags, droopy eyelids, and puffiness. Targeted Face Yoga exercises can strengthen and tone this muscle, reducing signs of aging and enhancing eye symmetry.

Why Strengthen the Orbicularis Oculi?

- Lifts droopy eyelids and prevents hooding
- Reduces crow's feet and fine lines around the eyes
- Diminishes dark circles and puffiness by improving lymphatic drainage
- Enhances eye symmetry, making the eyes look brighter and more open

1. Eye Opener Exercise

This exercise strengthens the orbicularis oculi and lifts sagging eyelids, making the eyes look more awake.

How to Perform:

1. Place index fingers under each eyebrow, gently lifting the skin upward.
2. Try to close your eyes slowly while keeping the brows lifted.
3. Hold the position for 5 seconds, then relax.
4. Repeat 10 times for best results.

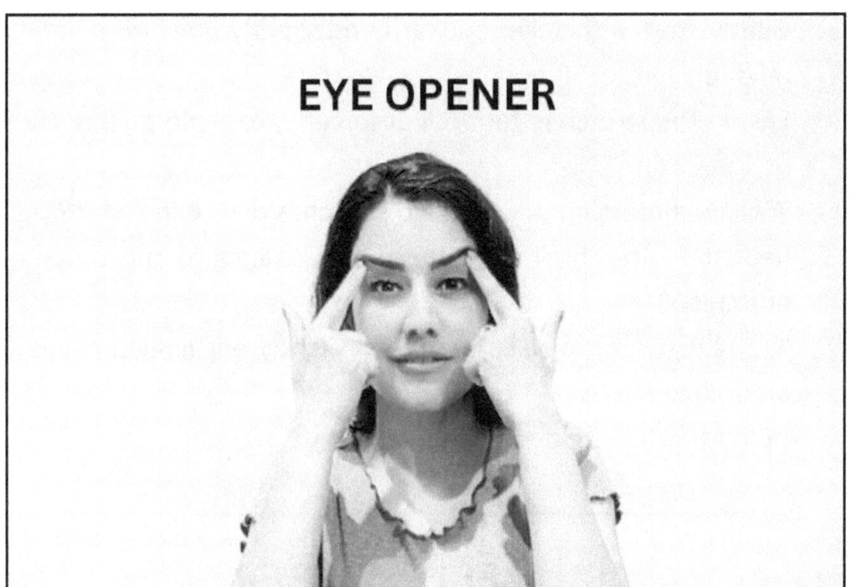

Benefits:

- Lifts drooping eyelids naturally
- Strengthens the upper eye muscles
- Improves eye openness and prevents hooded eyes

2. The Crow's Feet Smoother

The Crow's Feet Smoother exercise is designed to target fine lines and wrinkles around the outer corners of the eyes, commonly known as crow's feet. This technique stretches, strengthens, and massages the delicate skin around the eyes, promoting smoother skin, better circulation, and reduced puffiness.

How to Perform

1. Stretching the Outer Eye Area
2. Place your index and middle fingers of both hands on the outer corners of your eyes.

3. Gently stretch the skin outward and slightly upward, creating a mild tension.
4. Ensure the stretch is gentle, not forceful, to avoid pulling on the delicate skin.
5. While maintaining the outward stretch, slowly blink your eyes.
6. Repeat 5 slow blinks, feeling the resistance in the outer eye muscles.
7. Keep the stretch in place and squint slightly, engaging the muscles around your eyes.
8. Hold for 5-10 seconds, then release.

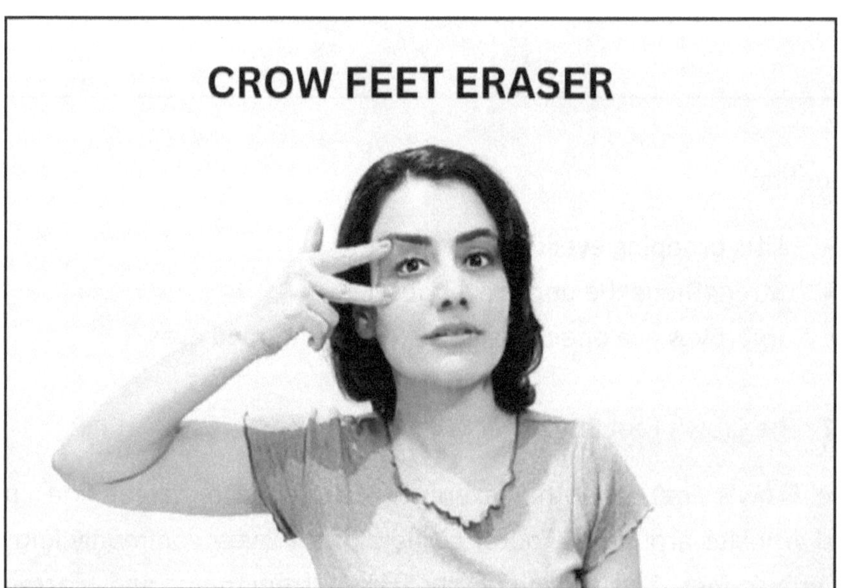

Benefits:

-   Prevents and reduces crow's feet by gently stretching the outer eye area
-   Boosts circulation to the inner eye, reducing puffiness and dark circles
-   Strengthens the orbicularis oculi muscle, preventing sagging

- Encourages lymphatic drainage to eliminate toxins and fluid retention
- Relaxes tension from squinting and eye strain

3. The Under-Eye Firmer (Reduces Puffiness & Dark Circles)

This technique activates the lower orbicularis oculi muscle, helping to reduce under-eye bags and dark circles.

How to Perform:

1. Place both index fingers under the eyes along the orbital bone.
2. Look upwards, then try to lift the lower eyelids without moving the upper eyelids.
3. Hold for 5 seconds, then relax.
4. Repeat 10 times.

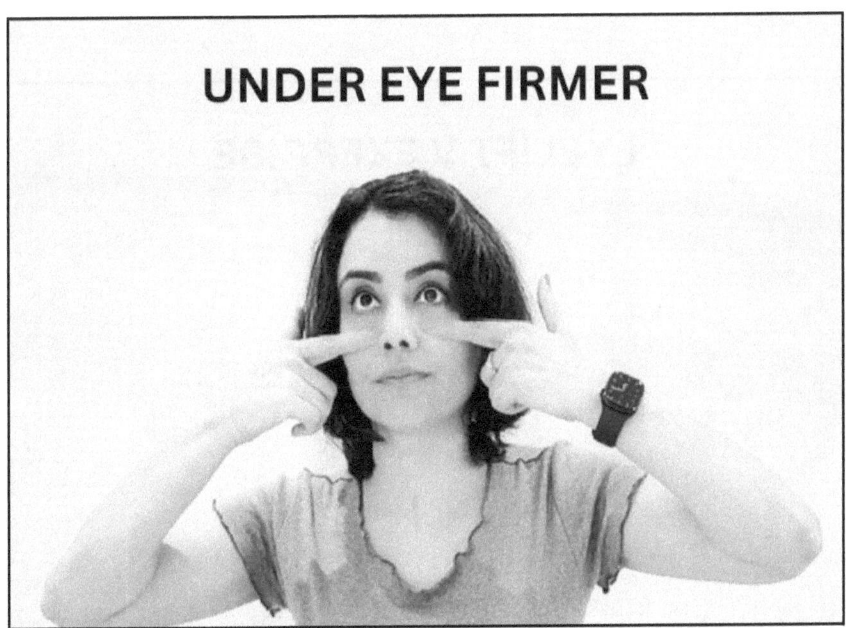

Benefits:

- Reduces puffiness and fluid retention
- Strengthens the lower eyelid, preventing eye hollowness
- Improves blood circulation to the under-eye area

4. The Eye Lift V Exercise

A powerful eye-lifting technique that helps maintain firm, youthful eyes.

How to Perform:

1. Place both middle fingers at the inner corners of the eyebrows.
2. Place both index fingers at the outer corners of the eyes.
3. Apply gentle resistance while trying to lift the lower eyelids.
4. Hold for 5 seconds, then relax.
5. Repeat 10 times.

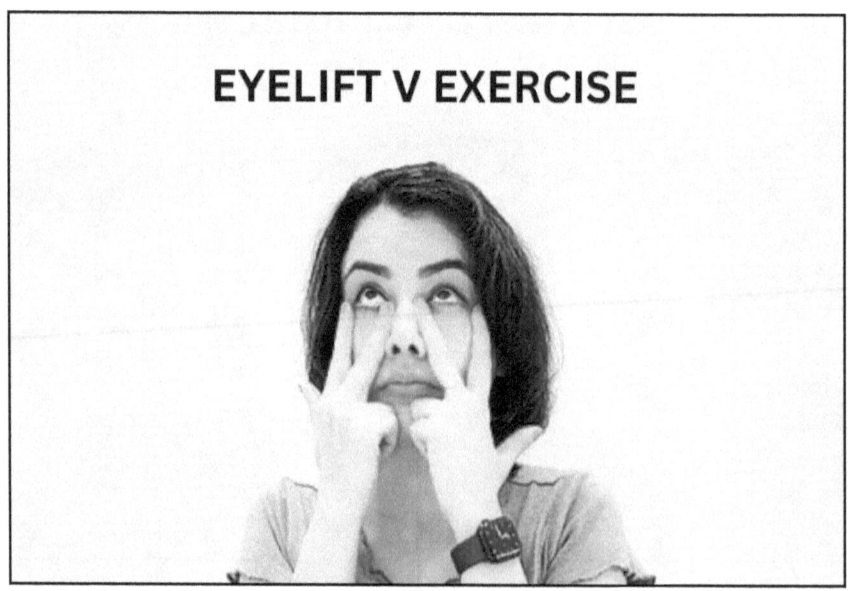

Benefits:

- Lifts sagging upper eyelids
- Reduces wrinkles at the outer eye corners
- Strengthens the entire eye area for a youthful look

5. The Eye Brightener

This stimulating exercise boosts blood flow and lymphatic drainage, helping to refresh tired eyes.

How to Perform:

1. Use both index fingers to gently tap around the entire eye socket, moving from the inner corner to the outer corner.
2. Continue tapping for 30 seconds while taking deep breaths.
3. Finish by gently pressing the temples and releasing tension.

Benefits:

- Reduces dark circles and under-eye puffiness
- Stimulates circulation for brighter eyes
- Relaxes the orbicularis oculi for a refreshed look

6. The Blinking Resistance Exercise

A resistance-based exercise that firms the orbicularis oculi, enhancing eye definition.

How to Perform:

1. Gently close your eyes halfway.
2. Hold this position for 5 seconds, feeling a slight resistance.
3. Slowly close your eyes fully and relax.
4. Repeat 10 times.

Benefits:

- Strengthens the eyelids and prevents sagging
- Enhances muscle control and eye firmness
- Reduces eye strain and fatigue

7. Flirty Owl Face Yoga Exercise

The Flirty Owl is a well-known Face Yoga exercise that targets the orbicularis oculi, frontalis, and corrugator supercilii muscles. It helps to lift the eyebrows, open the eyes, and smooth out forehead wrinkles. This exercise is excellent for reducing droopy eyelids, frown lines, and crow's feet, giving the eyes a more youthful and alert appearance.

How to Perform:

1. Place your thumbs on your Cheekbone and your index fingers just above your eyebrows, creating a "binocular" or "owl eyes" shape with your fingers.
2. Apply light pressure with your fingers and gently lift your eyebrows upward, creating resistance.
3. Open eyes as wide as possible, like you're surprised, without raising your eyebrows too much.
4. Try to hold your forehead smooth—avoid creating wrinkles.
5. Keep this position for 5-10 seconds, focusing on engaging the eye and forehead muscles.
6. Relax and repeat the exercise 5-10 times for best results.

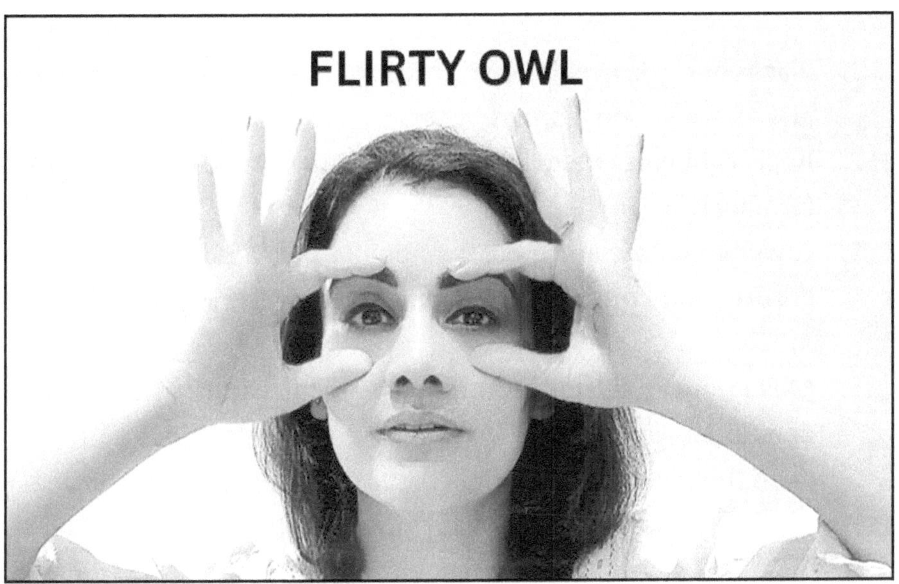

Benefits:

- Lifts droopy eyelids and prevents hooded eyes
- Reduces forehead wrinkles by training the frontalis muscle
- Strengthens the orbicularis oculi, improving eye shape
- Smooths frown lines between the brows
- Enhances blood circulation, making the eyes look brighter and more youthful

8. Pendulum Eye Exercise

This exercise helps release forehead tension, reduce eyestrain, and improve eye muscle flexibility. The controlled pendulum motion of the eyes, combined with forehead stabilisation, prevents unnecessary forehead movement and promotes relaxation.

How to Perform:

1. Place your index, middle and little fingers gently on your forehead, just above your eyebrows.
2. Apply light pressure to keep the forehead still and prevent wrinkle formation.
3. Lower your gaze and focus on a point downward.
4. Ensure your forehead remains relaxed, with no tension in the brows.
5. Move your eyes slowly from left to right and right to left in a pendulum-like motion.
6. Keep the movement controlled and smooth, without straining.
7. Avoid excessive blinking or squinting.
8. Close your eyes for a few seconds and blink rapidly 10 times to refresh them.

Repetitions:

- Perform 2–3 sets of 10 reps in each direction.

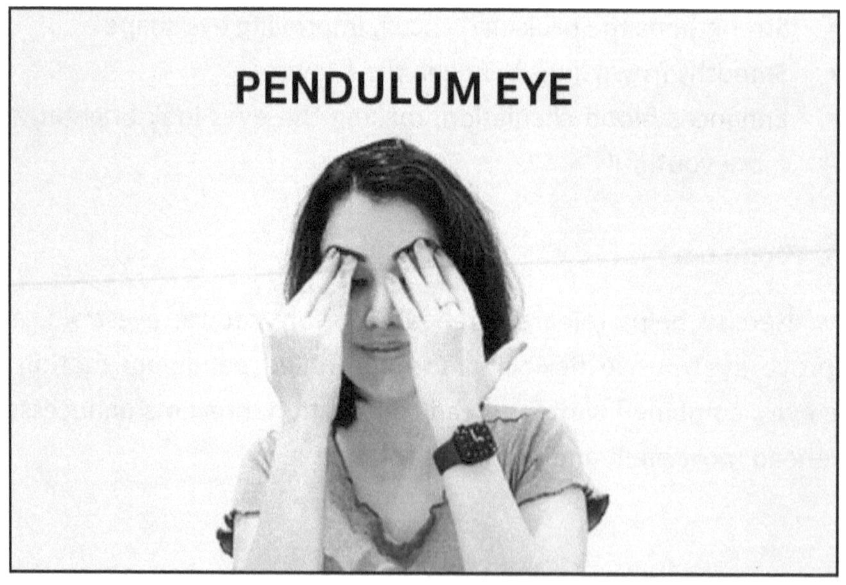

Benefits:

- Releases forehead tension and prevents wrinkles
- Strengthens eye muscles and reduces strain
- Improves eye flexibility and focus
- Encourages forehead relaxation, preventing frown lines

This exercise is perfect for screen users and those who frequently hold tension in the forehead.

Adding massage techniques can further enhance the effects of Face Yoga.

9. Droopy Eye Lifter Exercise

This enhanced exercise effectively lifts droopy eyelids, strengthens the levator muscles, and improves blood circulation, giving the eyes a more open and youthful look.

How to Perform:

1. Place one hand fingertips firmly on your eyelid to stabilize, lift and prevent unwanted movements.
2. With the fingertips of the other hand, tap the upper eyelid.
3. Make sure not to pull too hard—just enough to create slight resistance.
4. Continue tapping for 20–30 seconds to stimulate circulation.
5. After tapping, keep your eyelid lifted and try to blink slowly and deliberately 10 times.
6. Then relax your eyelid and repeat for 2–3 sets.

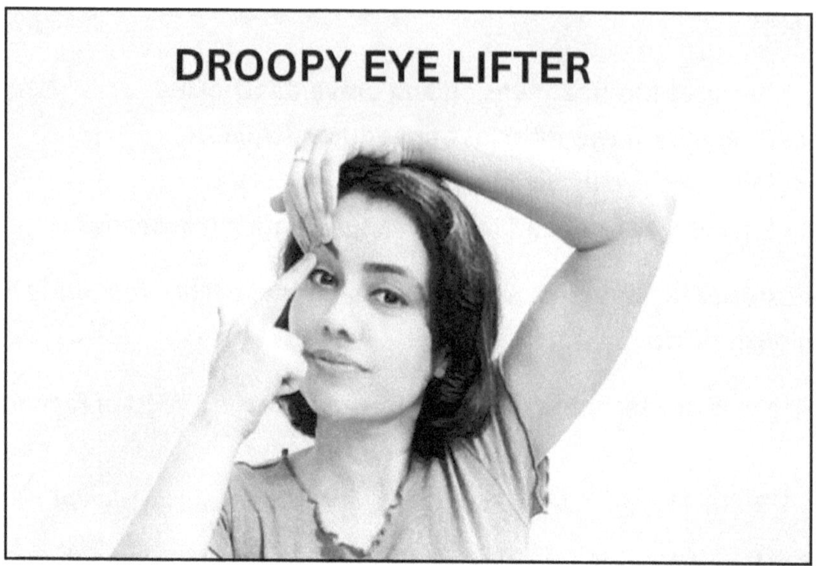

Benefits:

- Lifts and strengthens upper eyelid muscles
- Prevents sagging and drooping
- Enhances blood circulation for brighter eyes
- Reduces fatigue and signs of aging

10. Sucker Punch

This powerful eye-lifting exercise energises tired eyes, improves circulation, and helps firm the eye sockets by using warmth, vacuum pressure, and resistance.

How to Perform:

1. Rub your palms together vigorously for 5–10 seconds to generate warmth and energy.
2. Feel the heat building up in your hands.
3. Gently place your warm palms over your closed eyes, covering them completely.

4. Let the warmth relax your eye muscles for a few seconds.
5. Apply slight suction pressure by pressing your palms gently around your eye sockets.
6. Hold this position and slowly pull your hands outward, creating a subtle vacuum effect.
7. Maintain this gentle lift for 5 seconds before releasing.
8. Perform this 5–7 times in a controlled, rhythmic manner.
9. After the last round, open your eyes wide and blink rapidly 10 times to activate circulation.

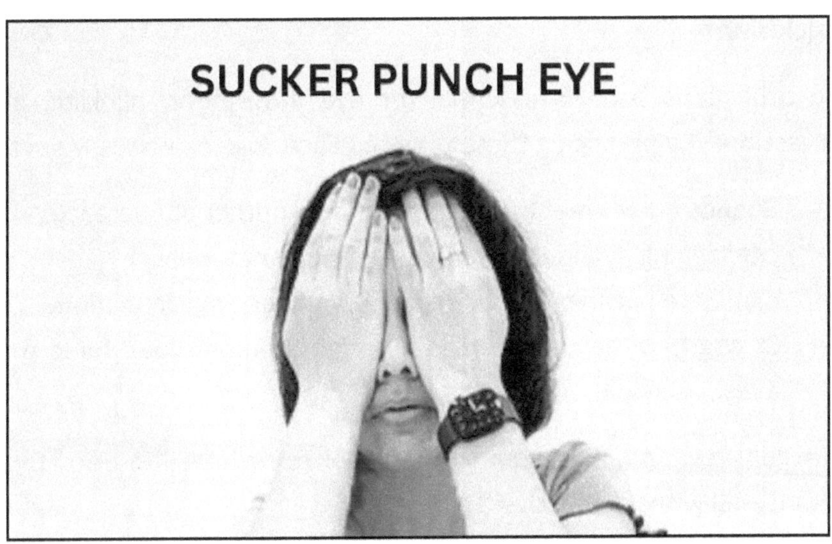

Benefits:

- Reduces eye tension and fatigue
- Lifts and firms the eye area
- Stimulates blood flow and brightens the eyes
- Helps reduce puffiness and dark circles

Key Tips for Effective Face Yoga for the Eyes

- Practice Daily: Consistency leads to visible results.
- Avoid Excessive Squinting: Wear sunglasses to prevent fine lines from sun exposure.
- Stay Hydrated: Drink plenty of water to keep the skin plump.
- Use Gentle Movements: The eye area is delicate, so apply minimal pressure.
- Combine with a Healthy Diet: Eating foods rich in vitamin C and antioxidants helps maintain firm skin.

Conclusion

The orbicularis oculi is essential for eye movement, blinking, and expressions. By practicing these targeted Face Yoga exercises, you can:

- Reduce crow's feet & fine lines for a smoother appearance.
- Lift sagging eyelids & improve eye shape naturally.
- Eliminate puffiness & dark circles by enhancing circulation.
- Strengthen the eye muscles for brighter, more youthful-looking eyes.

With consistent practice, your eyes will look refreshed, lifted, and more vibrant—all without invasive treatments!

Eye Tension Release Exercises

These exercises help relieve strain, relax the eye area, and reduce wrinkles caused by stress and screen time. They also improve circulation and lymphatic drainage for brighter, refreshed eyes.

1. Eye Palming (Warmth Relaxation)

How to Do It:

1. Rub your palms together to generate warmth.
2. Gently cup your palms over your closed eyes without pressing.
3. Breathe deeply and relax for 30 seconds to 1 minute.

Benefits: Relieves eye strain and promotes deep relaxation.

2. Eye Acupressure Points Release

How to Do It:

1. Use your ring fingers to gently press on these points for 5 seconds each:

   - Inner corner of the eyebrows
   - Middle of the eyebrows
   - Outer edge of the eyebrows
   - Temples

2. Repeat the cycle 2–3 times.

Benefits: Releases tension, reduces puffiness, and stimulates circulation.

3. Blinking & Eye Rolling (Muscle Relaxation)

How to Do It:

1. Blink 10 times rapidly to refresh the eyes.
2. Then, roll your eyes in a circular motion 5 times clockwise, then 5 times counterclockwise.

Benefits: Relieves digital eye strain and enhances eye mobility.

4. Pinch & Glide for Eyebrow Release

How to Do It:

1. Lightly pinch along the eyebrow from the center outwards.
2. Then, use your index and middle fingers to glide from under the eyes towards the temples for drainage.
3. Repeat 5 times.

Benefits: Releases tension, smooths fine lines, and promotes lymphatic flow.

5. Eye Stretch & Focus Reset

How to Do It:

1. Stretch your eyes wide open for 5 seconds, then relax.
2. Focus on a near object for 5 seconds, then shift to a far object for 5 seconds.
3. Repeat this cycle 5 times.

Benefits: Strengthens eye muscles and improves focus.

How Often?

- Daily practice helps prevent wrinkles, reduce puffiness, and relax eye muscles.
- Best done morning and night, or after long screen exposure.

In the next chapter, we will explore Face Yoga techniques for the cheeks, helping to lift, firm, and sculpt the mid-face area. Let's continue sculpting a naturally youthful face—one exercise at a time!

Cheeks Exercises

The cheeks play a crucial role in facial symmetry, youthfulness, and expression. Over time, factors like aging, gravity, and muscle loss can cause cheek sagging, nasolabial folds (smile lines), and loss of volume. Face Yoga exercises help strengthen, sculpt, and lift the cheek muscles, giving the face a firmer, fuller, and more youthful appearance.

Understanding the Cheek Muscles

Several key muscles contribute to the shape and tone of the cheeks:

- Zygomaticus Major & Minor – Lifts the cheeks and creates a youthful smile
- Buccinator – Supports cheek fullness and prevents hollowing
- Masseter – A jaw muscle that, when relaxed, reduces tension and slims the lower face
- Risorius – Helps with cheek definition and prevents sagging

By strengthening these muscles, Face Yoga helps to naturally lift, firm, and sculpt the cheeks, reducing sagging and enhancing facial harmony.

1. The Balloon Cheek

How to Perform:

1. Take a deep breath and puff up your cheeks, holding the air inside.
2. Slowly move the air from one cheek to the other (left to right) for 10 seconds.
3. Release the air and relax.
4. Repeat 3-5 times.

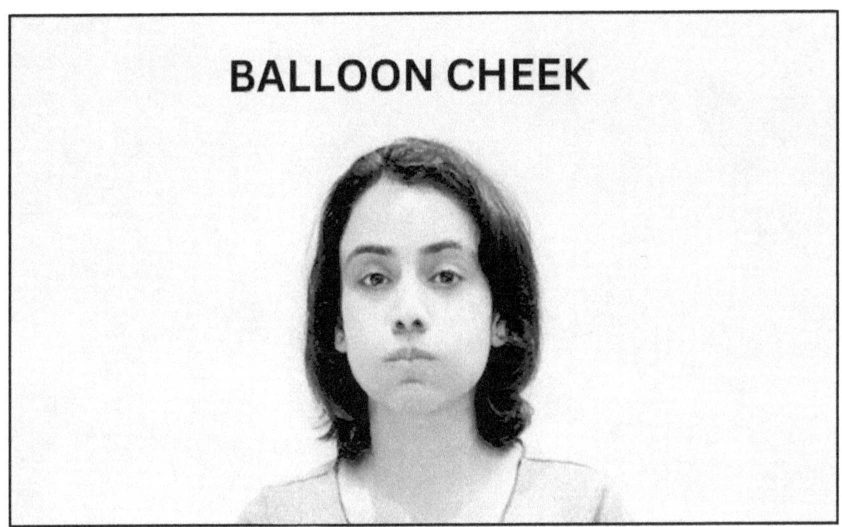

Benefits:

- Adds natural volume to the cheeks
- Strengthens buccinator muscles to prevent hollowing
- Improves blood circulation, giving a radiant glow

2. The Cheek Lifter

How to Perform:

1. Smile as wide as possible, engaging the cheek muscles.
2. Place your index fingers lightly on your cheekbones for support.
3. Gently lift your cheeks upward while supporting with your fingers.
4. Hold for 5-10 seconds, then relax.
5. Repeat 10 times.

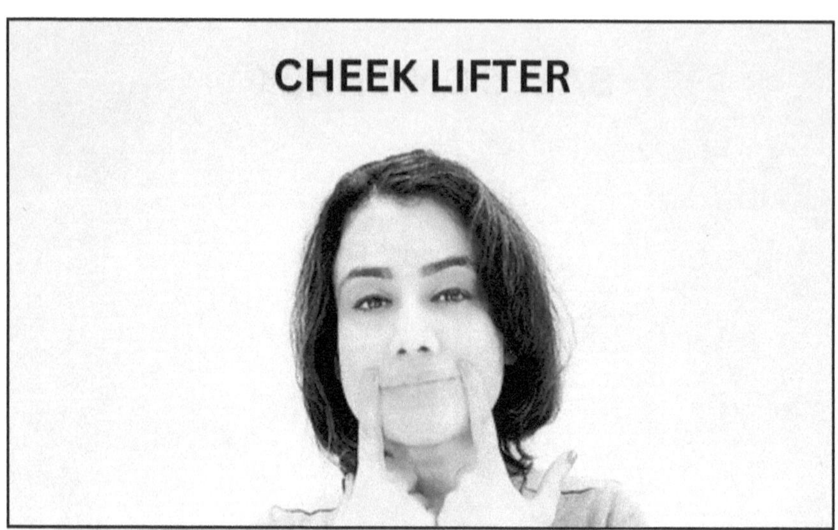

Benefits:

- Lifts and firms sagging cheeks
- Tones the zygomaticus major & minor muscles
- Prevents nasolabial folds and deep smile lines

3. The O-Smile

How to Perform:

1. Make an "O" shape with your mouth, covering your teeth with your lips.
2. Smile as wide as possible while keeping the lips over the teeth.
3. Hold for 10 seconds, feeling the cheek muscles engage.
4. Relax and repeat 10 times.

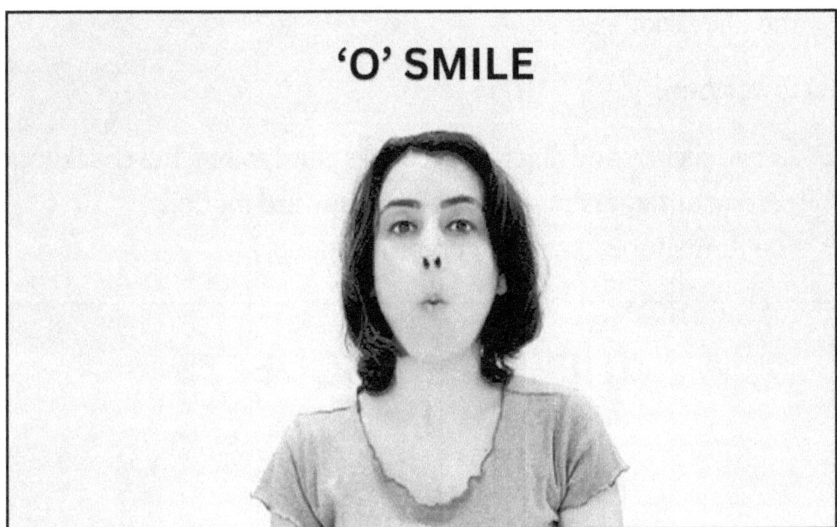

Benefits:

- Tightens the middle and upper cheek muscles
- Reduces deep smile lines and nasolabial folds
- Enhances cheek contour and definition

4. The Cheek Puff Resistance

How to Perform:

1. Puff out only one cheek and hold for 5 seconds.
2. Switch to the other cheek and hold for 5 seconds.
3. Puff out both cheeks together and hold for 10 seconds.
4. Repeat 3-5 times.

Benefits:

- Strengthens cheek muscles to maintain youthful fullness
- Increases collagen production, improving skin elasticity
- Prevents premature sagging and fine lines

5. The Cheekbone Squeeze

How to Perform:

1. Smile slightly and pinch your cheeks gently along the cheekbones.
2. Use your fingers to massage in an upward motion.
3. Continue for 30 seconds, breathing deeply.

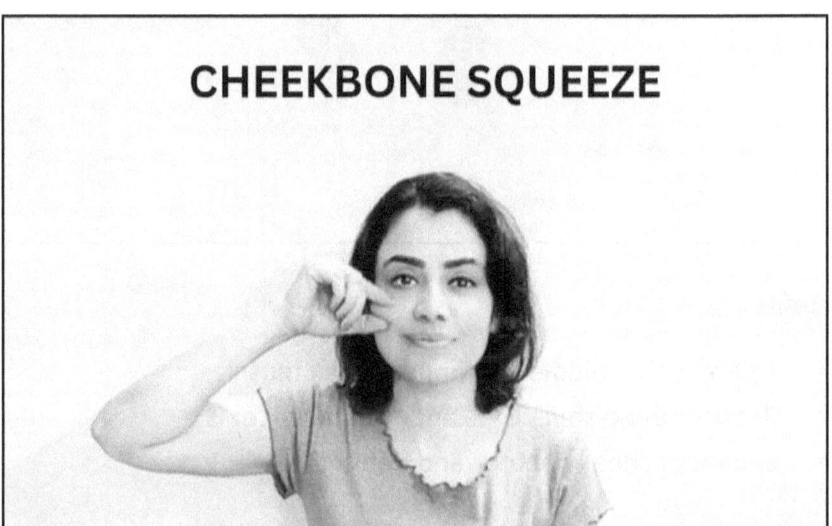

Benefits:

1. Enhances cheekbone definition
2. Stimulates collagen and circulation for a natural glow
3. Prevents sagging by lifting the muscles upward

6. The Spoon Lift

How to Perform:

1. Hold a spoon between your lips horizontally.
2. Lift the spoon upward using only your cheek muscles (not your lips).
3. Hold for 5 seconds, then lower it.
4. Repeat 5-10 times.

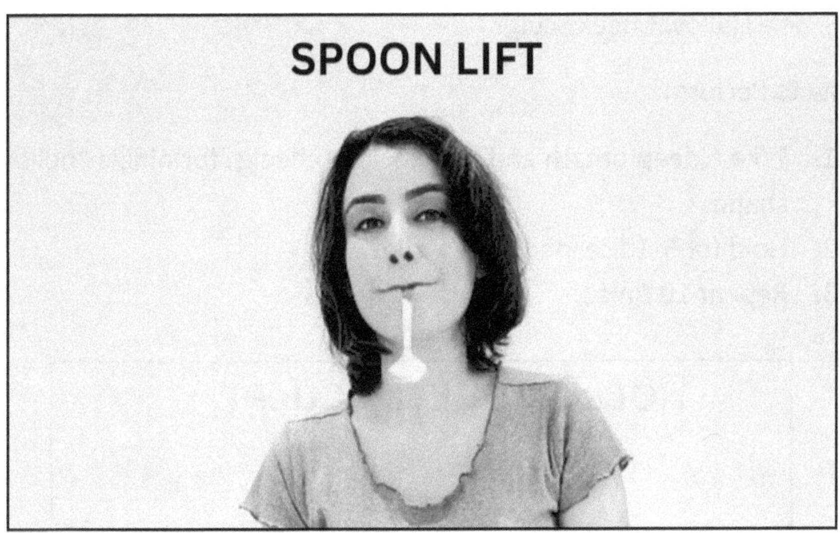

Benefits:

1. Strengthens zygomatic and buccinator muscles
2. Enhances cheek volume and firmness
3. Trains the cheeks to stay lifted naturally

7. The Kiss & Smile

How to Perform:

1. Pucker your lips as if you're blowing a kiss.
2. Now, smile widely while keeping your lips pursed.
3. Hold for 5 seconds, then relax.
4. Repeat 10 times.

Benefits:

- Strengthens cheek and lip muscles
- Prevents sagging of the lower cheek area
- Reduces laugh lines and lip wrinkles

8. The Hollow Cheek Sculpt

How to Perform:

1. Take a deep breath and suck in your cheeks, forming a "hollow" shape.
2. Hold for 5-10 seconds, then relax.
3. Repeat 10 times.

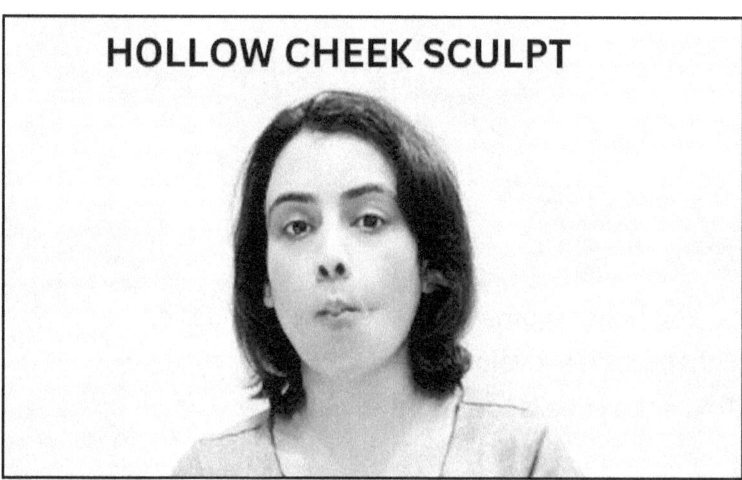

Benefits:

1. Highlights cheekbone prominence
2. Tones midface muscles for a sculpted effect
3. Supports natural facial structure

9. Face Squeezer

The "Face Squeezer" exercise is a rejuvenating face yoga technique that helps lift and sculpt the face by improving blood circulation, toning muscles, and reducing facial tension. This technique involves creating a triangle with your hands around your nose and using a massage motion to enhance lymphatic drainage and skin elasticity.

How to do Face Squeezer Exercise

1. Create a Triangle with Your Hands. Place your index fingers together at the bridge of your nose.
2. Position your thumbs under your chin, forming a triangle shape around your nose and mouth.
3. Press your fingers lightly along the sides of your nose.
4. Your thumbs should rest comfortably under your chin for support.
5. Slowly slide your fingers upwards along the sides of your nose, moving toward the temples.
6. Apply a gentle lifting motion as you go.
7. Focus on creating a smooth, upward movement to encourage skin elasticity.
8. Perform this movement 5-10 times in a slow, controlled manner.
9. Breathe deeply while massaging to enhance relaxation.

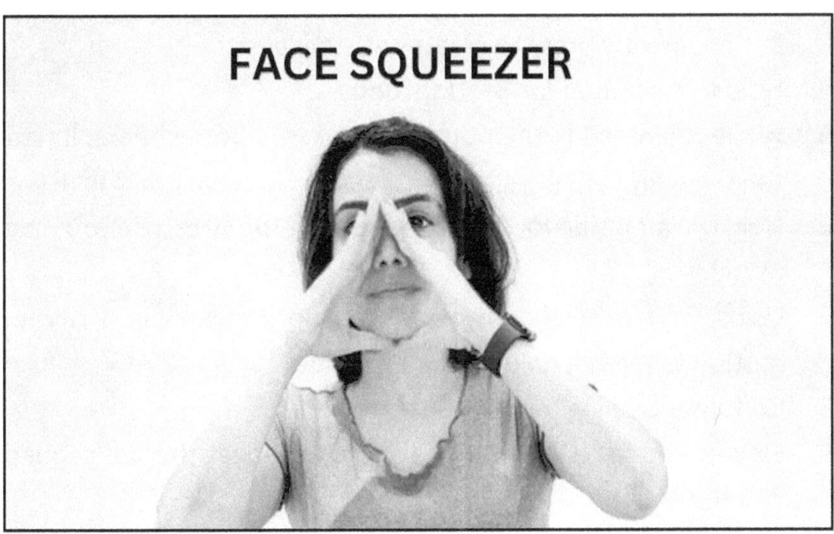

Benefits:

1. Lifts and sculpts the face naturally
2. Improves circulation, promoting a healthy glow

3. Reduces puffiness and enhances lymphatic drainage
4. Releases tension from facial muscles, especially around the eyes and cheeks
5. Tones and tightens the skin, minimising sagging

10. Cheek Lift & Air Resistance Exercise

This exercise tones and lifts the cheek muscles, improves circulation, and prevents sagging by combining lip resistance, air puffing, and tapping stimulation.

How to Perform:

1. Purse your lips forward into a tight pout, engaging your cheek muscles.
2. Keep your lips slightly tense and firm.
3. Place two fingers (index and middle fingers) over your pouted lips and gently press to create resistance.
4. Hold this position for 5–10 seconds.
5. While maintaining the pout, push air into both cheeks, inflating them evenly.
6. Hold the air inside for 5 seconds, feeling the stretch in your cheek muscles.
7. Using your other hand, gently tap both cheeks in a rhythmic motion while still holding the air inside.
8. Continue tapping for 10–15 seconds.
9. Slowly exhale, relax your cheeks, and repeat the full sequence 2–3 times.

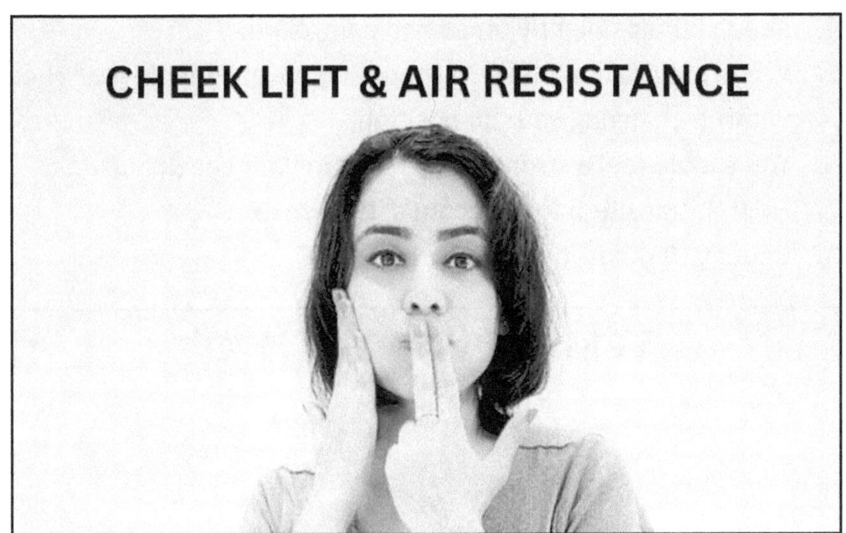

Benefits:

1. Lifts and strengthens the cheeks
2. Improves blood circulation for a youthful glow
3. Enhances cheekbone definition
4. Reduces sagging and fine lines

11. Temple Lift with O-Smile Exercise

This exercise helps lift the cheek muscles, define the jawline, and smooth nasolabial folds by combining resistance, muscle engagement, and stretching.

How to Perform:

1. Place both hands on your temples, with thumbs resting near your ears.
2. Apply a gentle upward lift with your hands to slightly stretch the skin.
3. Purse your lips into a small, tight "O" shape, engaging the muscles around your mouth.

4. Keep your lips slightly tense and controlled.
5. While maintaining the "O" shape, try to smile with your cheeks without changing your lip position.
6. You should feel a strong contraction in your cheek muscles.
7. Hold this position for 5 seconds, then relax.
8. Repeat 10 times for best results.

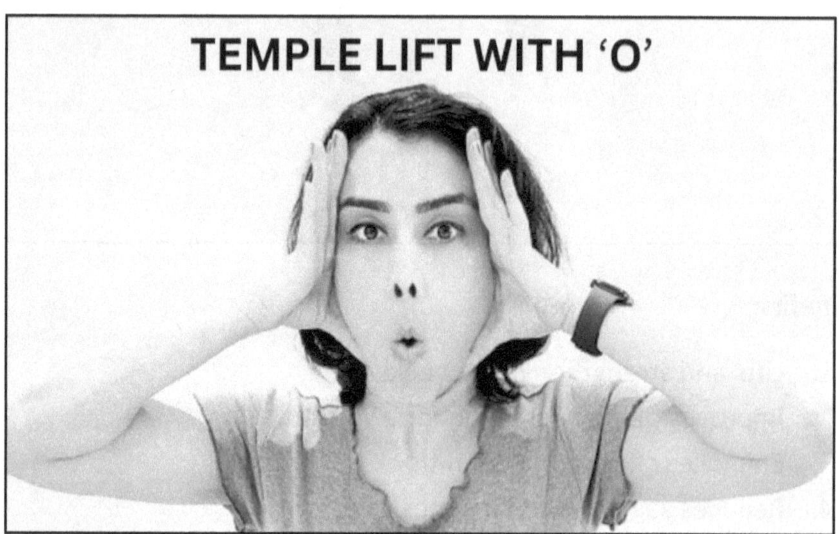

Benefits:

1. Lifts and sculpts the cheeks
2. Defines the jawline and smooths smile lines
3. Strengthens the mid-face muscles
4. Improves facial symmetry

12. Cheek Resistance with fist

This exercise helps lift and tone the cheeks, strengthen jaw muscles, and improve facial contour by using fist resistance while engaging the mouth and cheek muscles.

How to Perform:

1. Form a tight fist with both hands.
2. Place your knuckles against your cheeks, positioning them near the lower cheek area.
3. Press your fists into your cheeks, creating slight resistance.
4. Keep your elbows slightly bent and relaxed.
5. While maintaining the pressure from your fists, slowly open your mouth as wide as possible.
6. Feel the stretch in your cheeks and jaw muscles.

- Hold the open-mouth position for 5 seconds, then slowly close your mouth.
- Repeat 10 times in a slow, controlled motion.

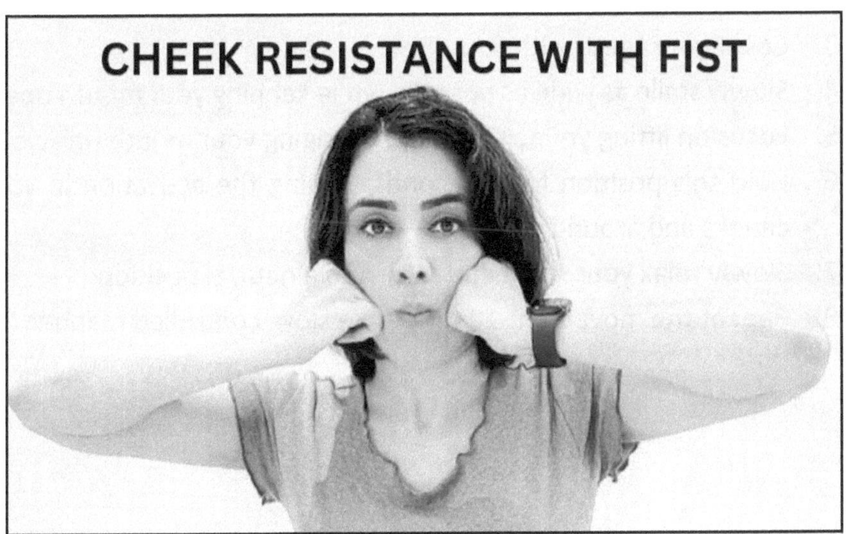

Benefits:

- Lifts and firms the cheeks
- Strengthens jaw and lower face muscles

- Improves cheekbone definition
- Helps reduce sagging and enhances facial symmetry

13. Open-Mouth Smile Exercise

This exercise helps lift the corners of the mouth, strengthen cheek muscles, and reduce nasolabial folds by combining resistance, controlled smiling, and muscle engagement while keeping the teeth covered.

How to Perform:

1. Place your index and middle fingers of both hands on either side of your lips, just above the corners of your mouth.
2. Apply gentle upward resistance, slightly lifting the skin toward your cheekbones.
3. Cover your teeth with your lips.
4. Slowly smile as wide as possible while keeping your mouth open.
5. Focus on lifting your cheeks and engaging your mouth muscles.
6. Hold this position for 5 seconds, feeling the activation in your cheeks and around your lips.
7. Slowly relax your smile and return to a neutral position.
8. Repeat the movement 10 times in a slow, controlled manner.

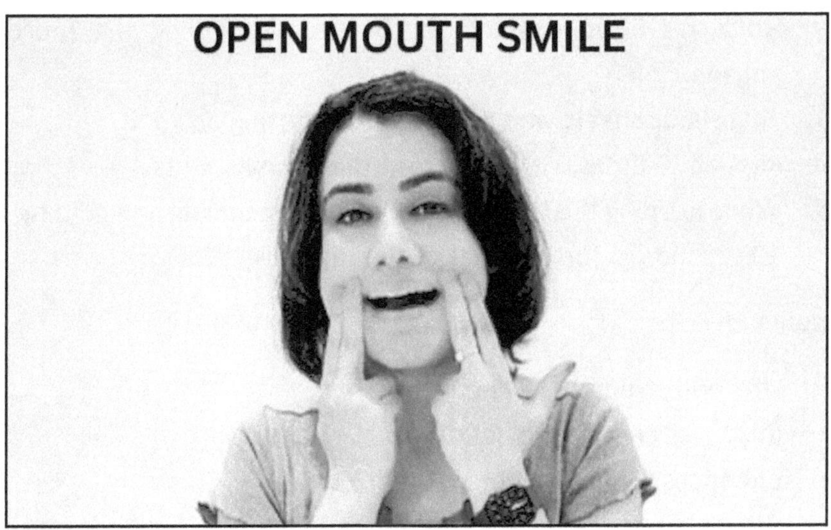

Benefits:

- Lifts and strengthens cheek muscles
- Defines the mouth and reduces nasolabial folds
- Tones the lower face and prevents sagging
- Improves facial symmetry and expression control

14. Cork Cap Cheek Lift Exercise

This exercise helps lift and tone the cheek muscles, strengthen the mid-face area, and improve facial symmetry by using a cork cap as resistance.

How to Perform:

1. Hold a cork cap gently between your lips
2. Keep your teeth slightly apart and avoid biting down—your lips and cheek muscles should do the work.
3. Slowly lift your cheek muscles upward, as if forming a big smile.
4. Keep the cork cap in place using only your lips and cheek strength.

5. Hold this lifted position for 5 seconds, feeling the muscles engage.
6. Relax your cheeks and return to the starting position.
7. Repeat 10 times with slow, controlled movements.
8. While keeping the cork in your mouth, try smiling and holding for 10 seconds to further engage the muscles.

Benefits:

- Lifts and strengthens cheek muscles
- Improves cheekbone definition
- Enhances facial symmetry and firmness
- Prevents sagging for a youthful appearance

15 The Cheek Massage & Lymphatic Drainage

How to Perform:

1. Apply a small amount of facial oil or moisturizer.
2. Use your fingertips to massage your cheeks in an upward motion, from the mouth toward the temples.
3. Perform gentle tapping motions along the cheekbones to stimulate blood flow.
4. Continue for 1-2 minutes daily.

Benefits:

- Enhances circulation and natural skin glow
- Releases tension and puffiness
- Helps tighten and tone the cheek area

Conclusion

The cheeks are one of the most expressive parts of the face, and maintaining their tone and structure is essential for a youthful, vibrant look. By incorporating these Face Yoga exercises, you can:

- Naturally lift and sculpt the cheekbones
- Reduce smile lines and sagging
- Enhance cheek fullness and definition
- Improve blood flow for a radiant, glowing complexion

In the next chapter, we will explore Face Yoga techniques for fuller lips. Let's continue sculpting a naturally youthful face—one exercise at a time!

Lips

Lips are a key feature of facial beauty and expression. Over time, aging, collagen loss, and muscle weakening can lead to thin lips, fine lines, and a loss of natural volume. Face Yoga exercises help to strengthen lip muscles, boost circulation, and enhance fullness naturally—without the need for fillers or invasive treatments.

Understanding Lip Muscles

Several muscles contribute to the shape and fullness of the lips:

- Orbicularis Oris – The primary muscle around the lips, responsible for lip movement and shape.
- Zygomaticus Major & Minor – Helps lift the corners of the mouth, preventing a downturned expression.
- Buccinator – Supports the sides of the lips and enhances volume.
- Depressor Anguli Oris – Affects the corners of the mouth, preventing sagging.

By strengthening and toning these muscles, Face Yoga helps to plump, define, and enhance lip shape naturally.

1. The Pout & Release

How to Perform:

1. Pucker your lips into a tight pout, as if you're about to kiss.
2. Hold this position for 5 seconds.
3. Slowly release and relax your lips.
4. Repeat 10 times.

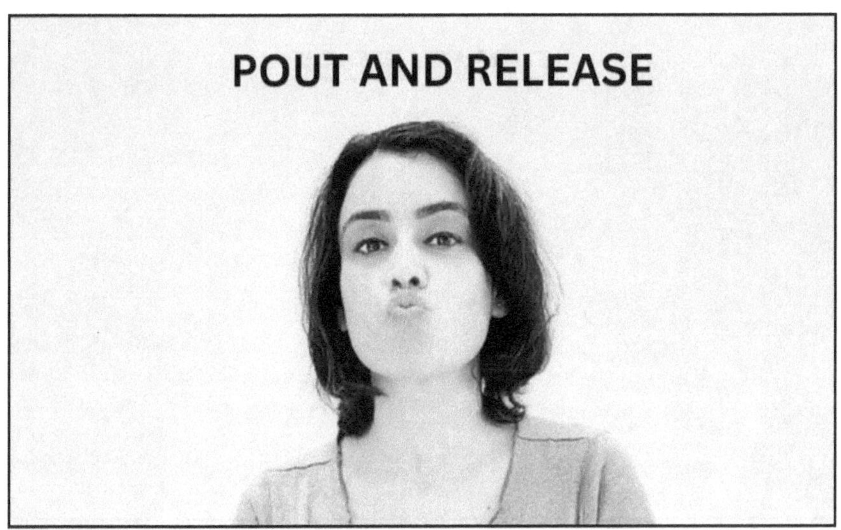

Benefits:

- Increases blood flow, making lips look naturally plumper
- Strengthens orbicularis oris for a defined lip shape
- Helps prevent lip thinning over time

2. Bumblebee

How to Perform:

1. Take a deep breath and blow air out through your lips while creating Vibration on lips.
2. Keep the airflow steady for 5-10 seconds.
3. Relax and repeat 10 times.

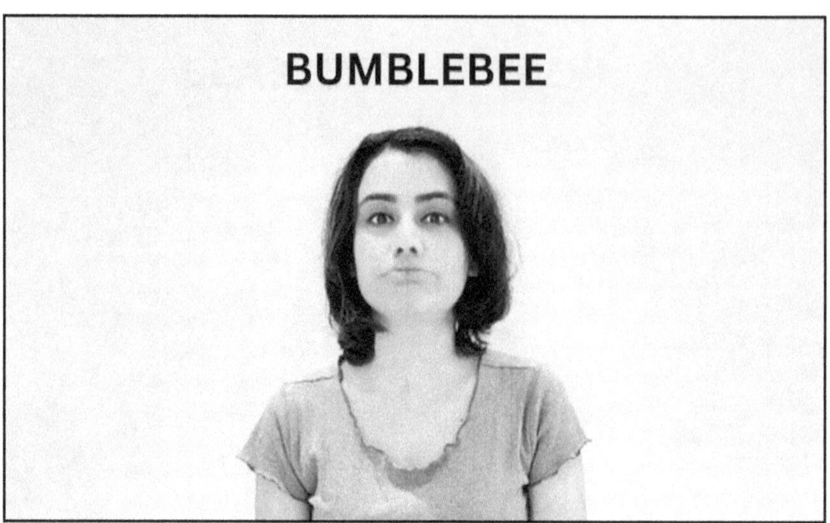

Benefits:

- Engages and tones the orbicularis oris muscle
- Boosts circulation for naturally pinker, fuller lips
- Strengthens lip muscles to prevent fine lines

3. The Smile & Kiss

How to Perform:

1. Smile widely without showing your teeth.
2. Now, pucker your lips into a kissing motion.
3. Hold each position for 5 seconds, then switch.
4. Repeat 10 times.

Benefits:

- Lifts the corners of the lips, preventing a downturned expression
- Strengthens lip muscles for improved firmness and fullness
- Reduces fine lines around the mouth

4. The Spoon Press

How to Perform:

1. Hold a spoon between your lips (horizontally).
2. Press your lips firmly around the spoon, engaging the lip muscles.
3. Hold for 5-10 seconds, then relax.
4. Repeat 5-10 times.

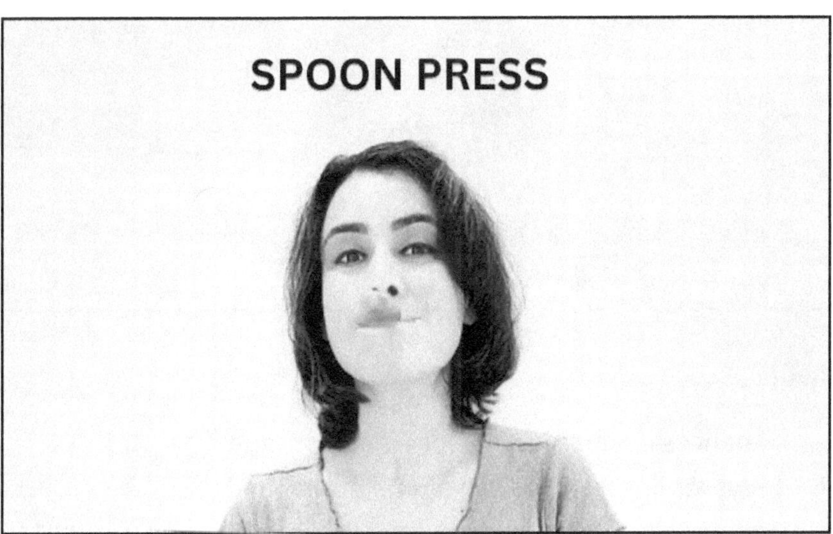

Benefits:

- Increases lip strength and fullness
- Tones the muscles around the lips for better definition
- Prevents lip wrinkles and sagging

5. The Lip Resistance Push

How to Perform:

1. Place two fingers on your lips, applying gentle resistance.
2. Try to purse your lips forward while pressing against your fingers.

3. Hold for 5 seconds, then relax.
4. Repeat 10 times.

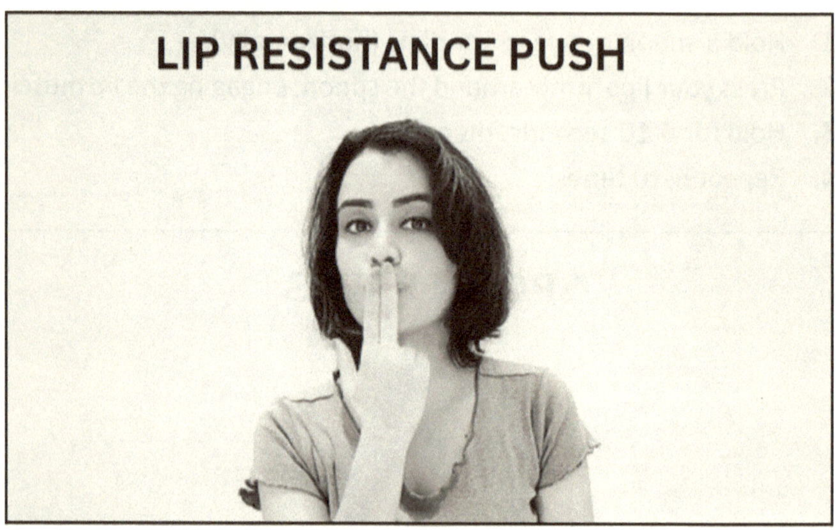

Benefits:

- Enhances lip muscle tone for a firmer shape
- Prevents lips from losing volume over time
- Boosts collagen production, keeping lips plump

6. The Lip Stretch

How to Perform:

1. Open your mouth slightly and stretch your lips over your teeth.
2. Try to smile while keeping your lips stretched.
3. Hold for 5 seconds, then relax.
4. Repeat 10 times.

Benefits:

- Strengthens lip and cheek muscles

- Reduces lip wrinkles and fine lines
- Enhances lip contour for a fuller appearance

7. The Finger-Tap Circulation Booster

How to Perform:

1. Use your fingertips to gently tap all over your lips.
2. Continue tapping for 30 seconds to stimulate circulation.
3. Relax and breathe deeply.

Benefits:

- Increases blood flow, giving lips a rosy, natural color
- Boosts collagen and oxygen supply for fuller lips
- Helps to smooth lip texture

8. Duck Lips

This advanced lip exercise helps plump, lift, and tone the lips while reducing fine lines around the mouth. The combination of pouting, fingertip resistance, and outward gliding enhances lip definition and stimulates blood circulation.

How to Perform:

1. Purse your lips forward into a tight pout as if you're about to kiss.
2. Keep the lips firm and engaged, feeling the muscles activate.
3. Hold the lips with both index fingers and thumbs from centre of your lips, lightly pressing down to create resistance.
4. While maintaining the pout, slowly glide your fingers outward toward the corners of your mouth.
5. Apply gentle but firm pressure as you move along the lips.
6. Repeat this gliding motion 10 times.

7. After the last glide, hold the stretched position for 5 seconds, then relax.

8. Repeat for 2–3 Sets. Perform the full exercise twice daily for best results.

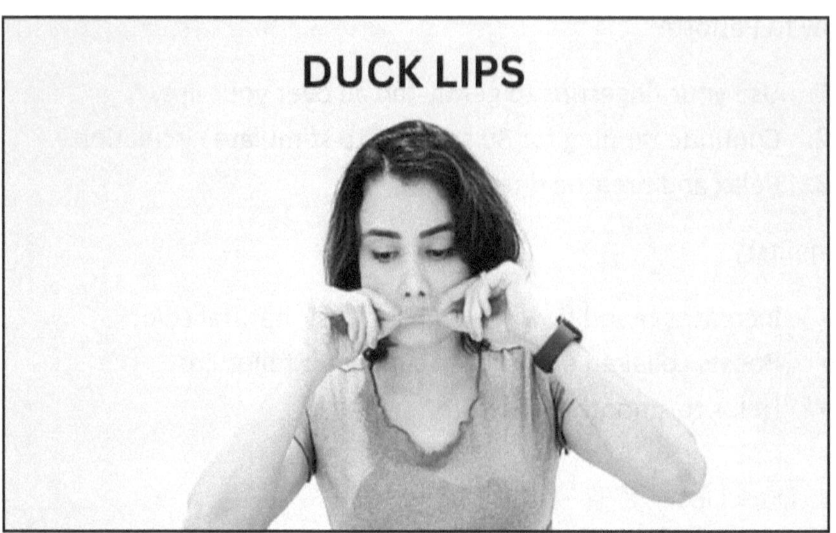

Benefits:

- Plumps and defines the lips naturally
- Reduces vertical lip lines
- Lifts and firms the lip corners
- Enhances blood circulation for a youthful glow

9. Little "O" Exercise

This exercise helps tone the orbicularis oris muscle, sculpt the jawline, and lift the lower face by engaging the lips and neck muscles. The upward gaze enhances the stretch, improving elasticity and reducing sagging.

How to Perform:

1. Purse your lips into a tight, small "O" shape.
2. Focus on bringing the corners of your lips as close together as possible.
3. Keep the lips slightly tense and engaged.
4. While maintaining the "O" shape, tilt your head back and look up toward the ceiling.
5. Feel a slight stretch along your chin, jawline, and neck.
6. Hold this position for 5–10 seconds, keeping the tension in your lips.
7. Breathe deeply through your nose while holding.
8. Slowly return to a neutral position.
9. Repeat 5–10 times for best results.

Benefits:

- Defines and lifts the lips
- Strengthens the jawline and neck muscles
- Improves lip symmetry and firmness
- Reduces sagging in the lower face

10. Lip Rotation Exercise

This exercise strengthens the orbicularis oris muscle, improves lip flexibility, and enhances circulation to create fuller, firmer lips while reducing fine lines around the mouth.

How to Perform:

1. Sit comfortably with your spine straight and shoulders relaxed.
2. Keep your forehead still to avoid tension.
3. Purse your lips forward into a gentle pout, engaging the muscles around your mouth.

4. Begin moving your lips in a circular motion, as if tracing a small invisible circle in the air.
5. Move in one direction for 10 slow rotations while keeping the movement controlled.
6. Then, switch directions and repeat 10 times in the opposite direction.
7. Keep your jaw still and only move your lips.
8. Ensure a smooth, steady rotation rather than quick, jerky movements.
9. Rest your lips for a few seconds and repeat the full sequence 2–3 times.

Benefits:

- Strengthens and defines lips
- Improves flexibility and symmetry
- Enhances blood flow for a natural rosy glow
- Helps reduce fine lines around the mouth

11. Lip Sumo Squat

This exercise helps strengthen the orbicularis oris muscle, improve lip definition, and enhance blood circulation, giving your lips a naturally plumper and firmer appearance. Inspired by a sumo squat, this movement involves controlled lip engagement and resistance.

How to Perform:

1. Purse your lips forward into a tight "O" shape, as if preparing to blow a kiss.
2. Keep your lips slightly tense and firm, engaging the surrounding muscles.
3. While keeping the "O" shape, pull your lower lip downward as if stretching it into a sumo squat stance.

4. Feel the stretch and engagement in your lip muscles.
5. Hold the stretched lower lip position for 5 seconds.
6. Then, pulse your lips up and down in small movements 10 times to activate the muscles further.
7. Relax your lips and return to the neutral position.
8. Repeat 10 times with controlled movements.

Benefits:

- Strengthens and defines lip muscles
- Increases lip volume naturally
- Improves circulation for a rosy glow
- Helps prevent lip thinning and fine lines

12. Lip Mobility Exercise

This exercise tones the jawline, strengthens the lower face muscles, and improves lip flexibility by using thumb resistance while moving the lips side to side.

How to Perform:

1. Place your thumb pads on the bottom of your jawline, just under your chin.
2. Apply gentle but firm pressure upward to create resistance.
3. Keeping your jaw still, slowly move your lips from left to right in a controlled motion.
4. Feel the muscles in your lower face engaging as you move.
5. Repeat the side-to-side lip movement 10 times.
6. Perform the motion slowly to maximize muscle engagement.
7. After the last repetition, hold your lips at each side for 3 seconds before switching.

Benefits:

- Strengthens jawline and lower face muscles
- Improves lip mobility and symmetry
- Enhances circulation for a youthful look
- Helps reduce sagging around the mouth and chin

13. The Lip Massage

How to Perform:

1. Apply a small amount of lip balm or oil.
2. Use your index and middle fingers to gently massage your lips in circular motions.
3. Continue for 1-2 minutes before bed.

Benefits:

- Hydrates and nourishes lips
- Increases blood circulation for natural volume
- Reduces tension and lip lines

Bonus Tips for Naturally Plump Lips

- Stay Hydrated: Dry lips appear thinner—drink plenty of water.
- Exfoliate Weekly: Use a lip scrub or a soft toothbrush to remove dead skin and boost circulation.
- Moisturize Daily: Use hyaluronic acid or shea butter lip balms to keep lips hydrated.
- Eat Collagen-Boosting Foods: Include vitamin C-rich foods to support natural plumpness.
- Avoid Smoking & Excessive Pouting: These habits create lip wrinkles and sagging.

Conclusion

Lips are a focal point of beauty, and maintaining their fullness, definition, and health is essential for a youthful appearance. By incorporating these Face Yoga exercises, you can:

- Naturally enhance lip fullness & shape
- Strengthen the muscles around the lips for a firmer look
- Reduce fine lines & prevent sagging
- Improve blood circulation for naturally pink, plump lips

With consistent practice, you'll achieve soft, lifted, and fuller lips—without injections or fillers!

In the next chapter, we will explore Face Yoga techniques for the nose. Let's continue sculpting a naturally youthful face—one exercise at a time!

Nose

The nose is a central feature of the face, and its appearance can change over time due to aging, gravity, and loss of muscle tone. While the bone structure of the nose cannot be altered without surgery, Face Yoga exercises can help tone, lift, and slim the nose by strengthening the muscles around it, improving circulation, and preventing sagging.

Understanding Nose Muscles

The nose is supported by small but essential muscles that influence its shape:

Nasalis Muscle – Controls nose width and nostril movement

- Procerus Muscle – Affects the bridge of the nose and helps prevent wrinkles
- Levator Labii Superioris – Lifts the sides of the nose, preventing drooping

Orbicularis Oris – Surrounds the mouth and influences the shape of the nose

By strengthening and toning these muscles, Face Yoga can create the illusion of a slimmer, more lifted nose over time.

1. The Nose Lift

How to Perform:

1. Place your index finger under the tip of your nose.
2. Gently push the tip of your nose upward.
3. Now, try to pull your upper lip downward, creating resistance.
4. Hold for 5 seconds, then relax.
5. Repeat 10 times.

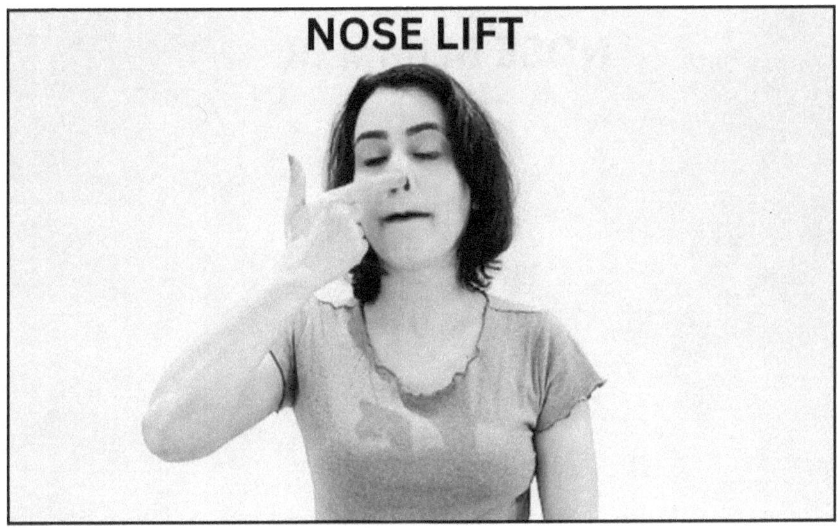

Benefits:

- Lifts the tip of the nose, preventing sagging
- Strengthens the nasalis and levator labii superioris
- Improves definition and shape of the nose

2. The Nose Slimmer

How to Perform:

1. Place your index fingers on the sides of your nose.
2. Apply gentle pressure while breathing deeply.
3. Hold for 5 seconds, then release.
4. Repeat 10 times.

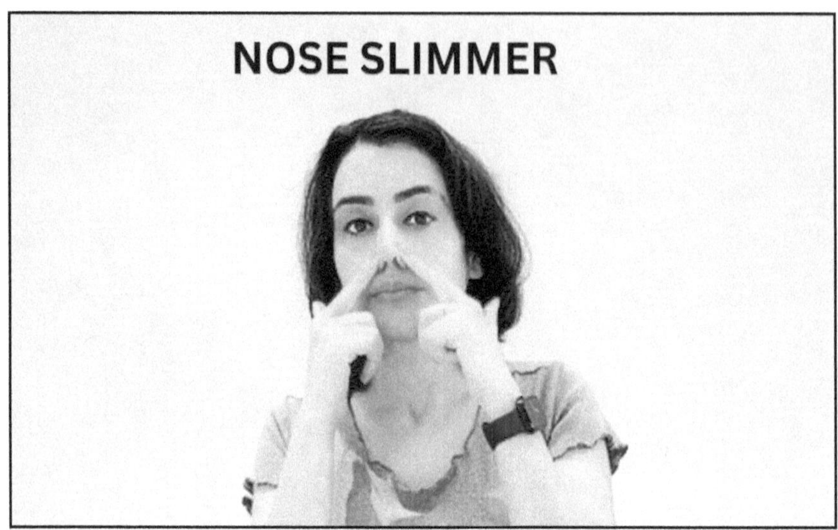

Benefits:

- Helps slim and define the sides of the nose
- Strengthens the nasalis muscle for better tone
- Enhances the nose's natural contour

3. The Procerus Smoother

How to Perform:

1. Place your index fingers between your eyebrows.
2. Apply gentle pressure and smooth the skin upward.
3. Hold for 5 seconds, then relax.
4. Repeat 10 times.

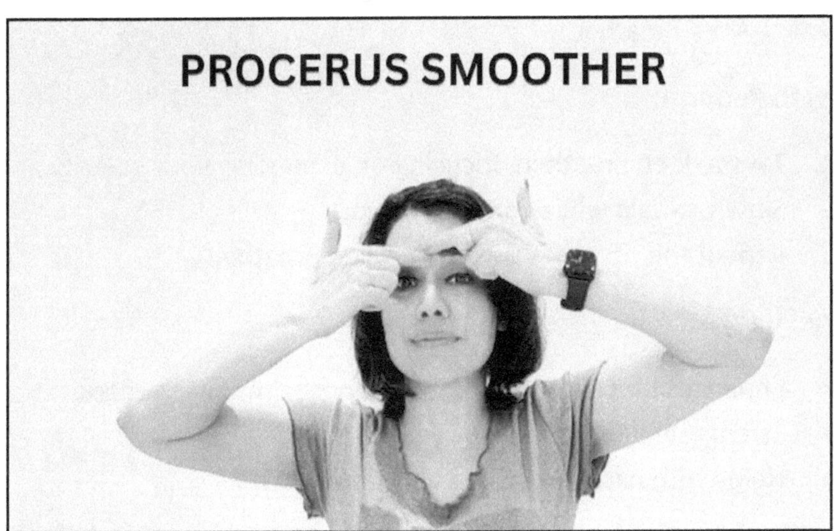

Benefits:

- Strengthens the procerus muscle, preventing nasal bridge wrinkles
- Creates a straighter, more refined nose bridge
- Reduces frown lines between the eyebrows

4. The Nose Wiggle

How to Perform:

1. Try to wiggle your nose from sides without moving your lips.
2. Focus on engaging your nasal muscles.
3. Continue for 30 seconds.

Benefits:

- Strengthens the nasal muscles for a firmer shape
- Improves muscle control and symmetry
- Helps define and tone the nose structure

5. The Nose Breather

How to Perform:

1. Take a deep breath in, focusing on expanding your nostrils.
2. Slowly exhale while contracting your nostrils.
3. Repeat this 10 times with controlled breathing.

Benefits:

*   Enhances blood circulation to the nose, improving shape
*   Strengthens the nasal muscles
*   Helps with nasal breathing and sinus health.

6. The Nose Pincher (For a More Defined Nose Tip)

How to Perform:

1. Pinch the tip of your nose gently using your thumb and index finger.
2. Hold for 5 seconds, then release.
3. Repeat 10 times.

Benefits:

*   Tones and firms the nasal tip
*   Helps maintain a lifted, defined shape
*   Prevents drooping of the nose tip with age

7. The Nose Massage

How to Perform:

1. Use your index fingers to massage the sides of your nose in an upward motion.
2. Continue for 30 seconds while breathing deeply.

Benefits:

- Stimulates lymphatic drainage, reducing puffiness
- Enhances blood circulation for a sculpted nose
- Helps prevent nasal sagging

Bonus Tips for a Naturally Sculpted Nose

- Stay Hydrated: Hydration helps prevent swelling and puffiness in the nose area.
- Maintain Good Posture: Poor posture can affect facial structure and make the nose appear different.
- Avoid Nose Rubbing: Repetitive pressure can alter the nasal structure over time.
- Use Facial Massage Tools: Jade rollers or gua sha can help contour the nose naturally.
- Breathe Correctly: Proper nasal breathing keeps the nose muscles active and toned.

Conclusion

While Face Yoga cannot change the bone structure of the nose, it can help to refine, lift, and tone the surrounding muscles, giving the appearance of a slimmer, more defined nose. By practicing these exercises regularly, you can:

- Prevent nasal tip drooping with age
- Strengthen the muscles for better nose tone
- Improve blood circulation for a more sculpted look
- Reduce puffiness and refine the nasal contours

With consistency and proper technique, you'll notice subtle yet effective changes in your nose shape, creating a more youthful, lifted appearance—naturally!

Neck

The neck is one of the first areas to show signs of aging, sagging, and wrinkles due to its delicate skin and muscle structure. Factors like poor posture, lack of muscle engagement, gravity, and decreased collagen production can lead to concerns such as turkey neck, horizontal lines, and skin laxity.

Face Yoga exercises help strengthen neck muscles, improve circulation, tighten skin, and enhance overall definition, creating a younger, firmer, and more toned neck appearance.

Understanding Neck Muscles. Several muscles contribute to the firmness, elasticity, and tone of the neck:

- Platysma – A broad sheet-like muscle responsible for lifting and tightening the neck and jawline.
- Sternocleidomastoid (SCM) – Extends from the jaw to the collarbone, contributing to neck elongation and firmness.
- Hyoid Muscles – Located at the front of the neck, crucial for supporting chin and throat contour.

By activating and strengthening these muscles, Face Yoga helps to sculpt, lift, and firm the neck naturally.

1. The Swan Neck Stretch

How to Perform:

1. Sit or stand with a straight back.
2. Turn your head to the right, looking over your shoulder.
3. Tilt your chin slightly upward, feeling a stretch in the side of your neck.
4. Hold for 5-10 seconds, then switch to the left side.
5. Repeat 5 times per side.

Benefits:

- Lengthens and tightens neck muscles
- Reduces horizontal lines and sagging
- Improves neck posture and flexibility

2. The Neck Lift

How to Perform:

1. Sit or stand with your spine straight.
2. Tilt your head backward, looking at the ceiling.
3. Pucker your lips as if you're kissing the ceiling.
4. Hold for 5-10 seconds, feeling a stretch in your neck.
5. Relax and repeat 10 times.

Benefits:

- Strengthens the platysma muscle
- Helps reduce turkey neck and sagging
- Improves neck firmness and elasticity

3. The Giraffe Stretch

How to Perform:

1. Sit or stand with a straight back.
2. Place your hands on your collarbone and apply slight downward pressure.
3. Tilt your head back and push your lower lip forward.
4. Hold for 5 seconds, then relax.
5. Repeat 10 times.

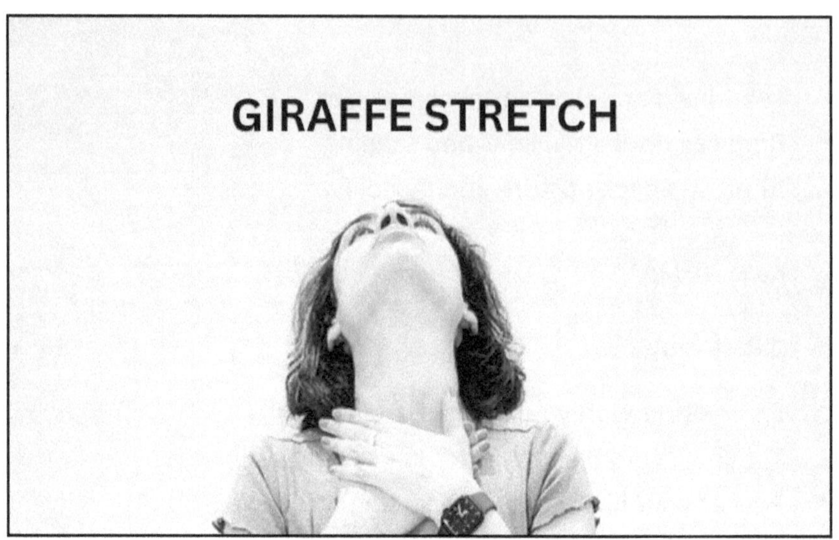

Benefits:

- Stretches and tones the front of the neck
- Improves skin firmness and elasticity
- Prevents neck wrinkles and sagging

4. The Neck Roll

How to Perform:

1. Sit upright with your shoulders relaxed.
2. Slowly tilt your head to the right, bringing your ear toward your shoulder.
3. Gently roll your head forward, bringing your chin to your chest.
4. Continue rolling to the left side, then back up.
5. Perform 5 slow rotations in each direction.

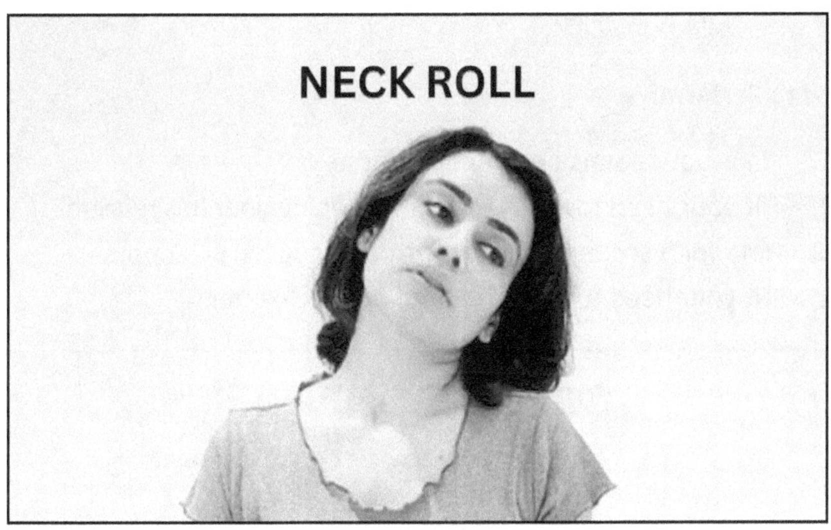

Benefits:

- Improves neck flexibility and circulation
- Reduces stiffness and horizontal lines
- Relieves tension and improves posture

5. The Tongue Press

How to Perform:

1. Sit with a straight spine.
2. Press your tongue against the roof of your mouth.
3. Tilt your head back slightly, feeling resistance in your neck.
4. Hold for 5 seconds, then relax.
5. Repeat 10 times.

Benefits:

- Strengthens neck and jawline muscles
- Reduces loose skin under the chin
- Enhances neck contouring

6. The Collarbone Lift

How to Perform:

1. Place your palms on your collarbone.
2. Tilt your head towards the right keeping your lips relaxed.
3. Hold for 5 seconds, then return to a neutral position.
4. Tilt your head towards left and back to center.

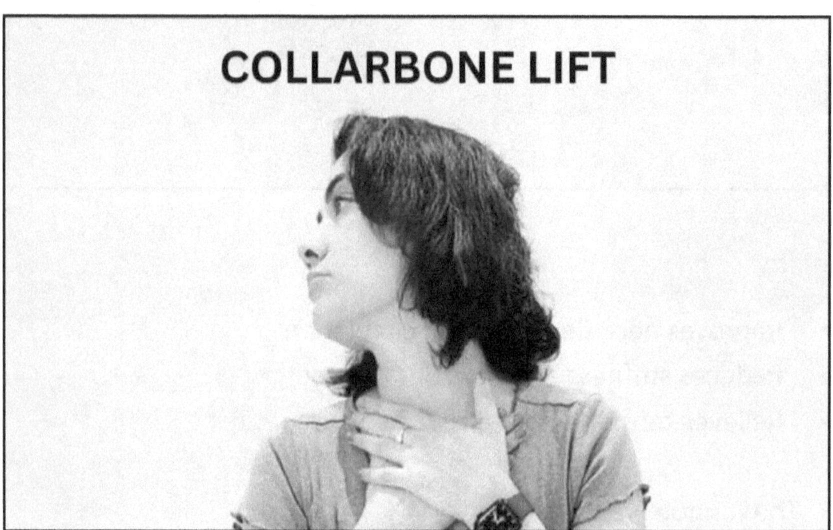

Benefits:

- Helps reduce fine lines and sagging
- Strengthens the platysma muscle
- Enhances neck elasticity

7. The Jaw Release

How to Perform:

1. Sit with a straight posture.
2. Slowly move your lower jaw right and left, keeping upper jaw stationary.

3. Hold the stretched position for 5 seconds, then relax.
4. Repeat 10 times.

Benefits:

- Tones neck and jawline muscles
- Improves neck definition and tightness
- Enhances jawline sharpness

Bonus Tips for a Toned Neck

- Stay Hydrated: Water helps keep neck skin firm and elastic.
- Practice Good Posture: Poor posture leads to neck wrinkles and sagging. Keep your head high and shoulders back.
- Avoid Looking Down at Phones (Tech Neck): Repeated downward movement creates horizontal neck lines. Hold your phone at eye level.
- Use Neck-Specific Skincare: Apply moisturizer, SPF, and collagen-boosting serums to maintain skin elasticity.
- Massage the Neck Regularly: Helps with lymphatic drainage, improves circulation, and prevents sagging.

By practicing these exercises daily, you can achieve a longer, firmer, and sculpted neck—naturally!

Chin and Jawline

The chin and jawline play a crucial role in facial structure, symmetry, and youthfulness. However, factors like aging, poor posture, excess fat, and muscle laxity can lead to double chin, sagging skin, and loss of definition.

Face Yoga offers natural and effective techniques to strengthen muscles, reduce excess fat, and tone the jawline and chin, helping you achieve a more defined and sculpted appearance.

Understanding Chin & Jawline Muscles

Several key muscles contribute to the firmness and definition of the chin and jawline:

- Platysma – A large muscle extending from the chin to the neck, responsible for jaw tightness.
- Digastric & Mylohyoid – Located under the chin, helping lift and support the jawline.
- Masseter – The primary chewing muscle, crucial for jaw strength and definition.
- Mentalis – Supports the chin and prevents dimpling or sagging.

One of the most effective natural techniques for enhancing your jawline is mewing—a method that involves proper tongue posture to shape and define the jawbone over time. Mewing exercises can help tone the jawline, improve facial symmetry, and even aid in breathing and posture.

In this chapter, we'll explore the science behind mewing, and step-by-step exercises to achieve a more sculpted jawline naturally.

What is Mewing? The Science Behind It

Mewing is a tongue posture technique that involves resting your tongue correctly against the roof of your mouth rather than letting it sit at the bottom. This practice, popularized by Dr. John Mew, is believed to improve jawline definition, reduce double chin, and enhance overall facial structure over time.

When practiced consistently, mewing helps to:

- Encourage proper jaw positioning
- Tone and tighten the jaw and chin muscles
- Reduce facial puffiness by improving lymphatic drainage
- Enhance breathing and posture

Results vary, but many people see improvements in their jawline within a few months of practicing mewing consistently.

Step-by-Step Guide to Mewing

- Close your mouth and ensure your teeth are lightly touching (not clenched).
- Press the entire tongue flat against the roof of your mouth (not just the tip).
- Your lips should be sealed but relaxed.
- Breathe through your nose, not your mouth.
- Mewing is a long-term practice; it won't give instant results but works over time.
- Keep your tongue in the correct posture throughout the day.
- Be mindful of your posture, as slouching can impact jawline definition.
- Combine Mewing with Jawline Exercises

1. The Jaw Jut

How to Perform:

1. Tilt your head slightly backward.
2. Push your lower jaw forward, creating tension in the chin.

3. Hold for 5 seconds, then relax.
4. Repeat 10 times.

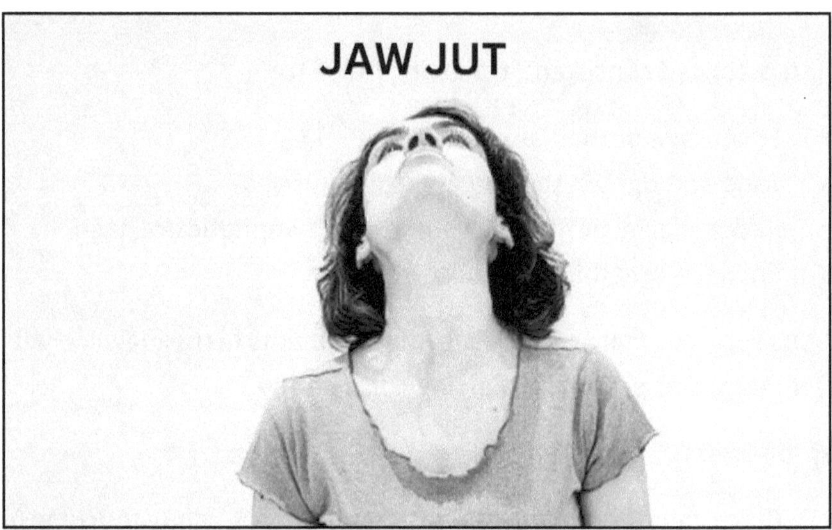

Benefits:

- Defines the chin and jawline
- Strengthens jaw muscles
- Reduces loose skin under the chin

2. The Chin Lift

How to Perform:

1. Sit or stand with a straight back.
2. Tilt your head backwards, looking at the ceiling.
3. Pucker your lips as if you're trying to kiss the ceiling.
4. Hold for 5-10 seconds, feeling a stretch in your chin and jawline.
5. Relax and repeat 10 times.

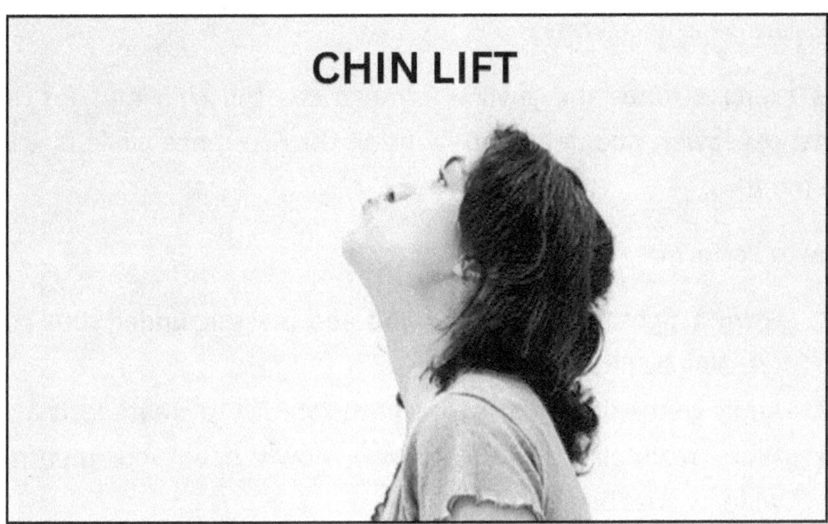

Benefits:

- Strengthens the platysma and mentalis muscles
- Reduces double chin and sagging
- Improves jawline definition

3. The Vowel Stretch

How to Perform:

1. Open your mouth wide and say "O" for 5 seconds.
2. Then say "E" while stretching your lips as much as possible.
3. Repeat both movements 10 times.

Benefits:

- Strengthens cheek and jaw muscles
- Enhances jawline definition
- Reduces sagging and wrinkles

4. Jaw Resistance Press

This exercise tones the jawline, strengthens the chin muscles, and enhances lower face definition by using fist resistance while opening the mouth

How to Perform:

1. Form a tight fist with one hand and place it under your chin, pressing against the lower jaw.
2. Apply gentle upward pressure with your fist to create resistance.
3. While maintaining the resistance, slowly open your mouth as wide as possible.
4. Feel the stretch and engagement in your jaw and chin muscles.
5. Hold the open-mouth position for 5 seconds, resisting against your fist.
6. Then slowly close your mouth, maintaining control.
7. Perform 10 slow, controlled repetitions.
8. For an advanced version, try pulsing your mouth slightly open and closed while maintaining fist pressure.

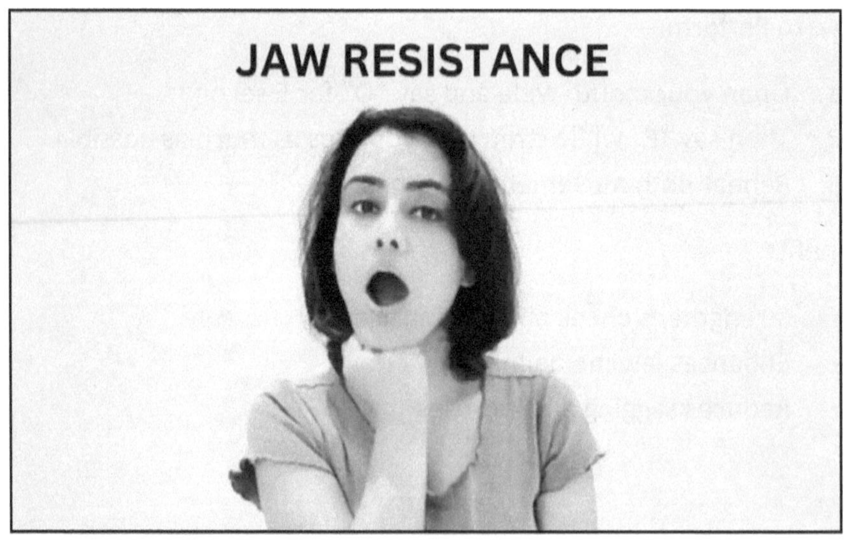

Benefits:

- Strengthens jaw and chin muscles
- Enhances jawline definition
- Reduces sagging and double chin appearance
- Improves overall facial symmetry

5. The Fish Face

How to Perform:

1. Suck in your cheeks and lips, creating a "fish face."
2. Try to smile while holding this position.
3. Hold for 5 seconds, then relax.
4. Repeat 10 times.

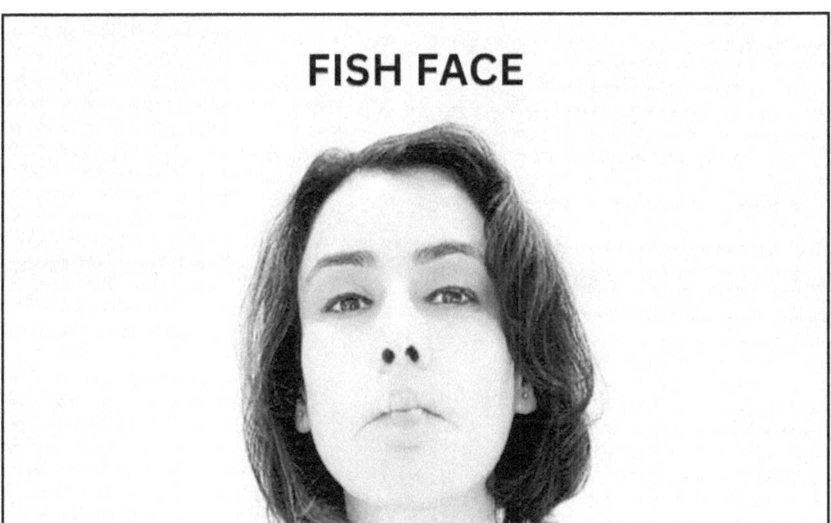

Benefits:

- Strengthens the jaw and chin muscles
- Helps slim the lower face
- Enhances jawline firmness

6. The Tennis Ball Squeeze

How to Perform:

1. Place a tennis ball under your chin.
2. Press your chin down firmly against the ball.
3. Hold for 5 seconds, then relax.
4. Repeat 10 times.

Benefits:

- Strengthens jaw and chin muscles
- Reduces double chin appearance
- Improves chin tightness

7. The Jawline Massage

How to Perform:

1. Apply a small amount of facial oil.
2. Use your fingers to massage in an upward motion from chin to jawline.
3. Continue for 1-2 minutes, focusing on tight areas.

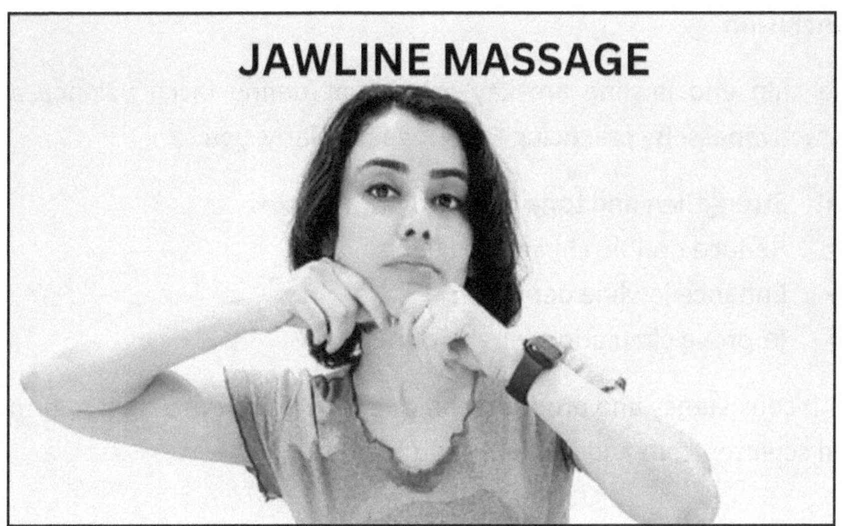

Benefits:

- Stimulates lymphatic drainage, reducing puffiness
- Enhances blood circulation for a youthful glow
- Firms the chin and jawline

Bonus Tips for a Sculpted Chin & Jawline

- Stay Hydrated: Keeps the skin firm and elastic.
- Maintain Good Posture: Slouching weakens jaw muscles; keep your head high and back straight.
- Avoid Excess Salt & Sugar: Too much salt leads to water retention and puffiness in the chin area.
- Eat Collagen-Rich Foods: Include bone broth, leafy greens, and vitamin C-rich foods to support skin elasticity.
- Use Sunscreen Daily: UV damage accelerates sagging and skin aging.

Conclusion

The chin and jawline are key areas that define facial balance and attractiveness. By practicing Face Yoga regularly, you can:

- Strengthen and tone chin and jaw muscles
- Reduce double chin and sagging
- Enhance jawline definition
- Improve circulation for a youthful glow

With consistency and proper technique, you'll achieve a tighter, firmer, and sculpted chin and jawline—naturally!

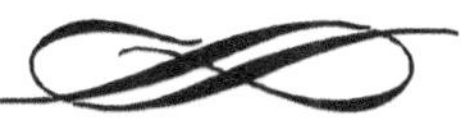

TMJ HEALTH TEST

Understanding the TMJ and Its Importance

The Temporomandibular Joint (TMJ) is one of the most crucial joints in the human body, allowing you to open and close your mouth for essential functions such as speaking, eating, and even breathing. When your TMJ is functioning properly, you won't experience discomfort or limitations in movement. However, when the TMJ is stiff, misaligned, or weak, it can lead to pain, tension, and even disorders such as TMJ dysfunction (TMD).

A simple test—**the Four-Finger Test**—can help you determine whether your TMJ is healthy or if it needs work.

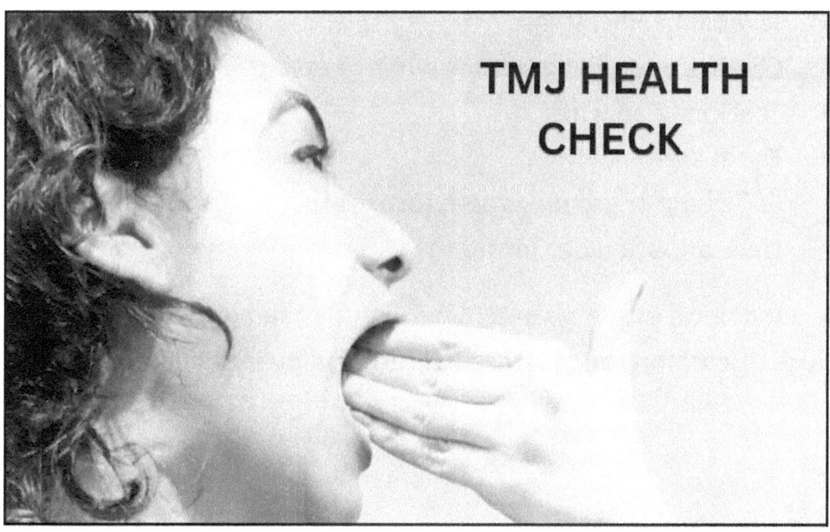

The Four-Finger Test: How to Check Your TMJ Health

- Sit in front of a mirror with a relaxed posture.
- Keep your head straight and your shoulders relaxed.
- Place your index, middle, ring, and pinky fingers of one hand together.
- Try inserting these four fingers vertically into your mouth, between your upper and lower teeth.

- If all four fingers fit comfortably → Your TMJ is healthy and functioning well.
- If only three fingers fit → You may have some mild TMJ tightness and should consider jaw mobility exercises.
- If only two fingers fit or you struggle with three → Your TMJ is significantly restricted, and you need targeted exercises to restore flexibility and strength.

Why Is Jaw Mobility Important?

A restricted TMJ can cause:

- Jaw pain and stiffness
- Clicking or popping sounds when chewing
- Tension headaches
- Facial asymmetry
- Clenching or grinding teeth (bruxism)
- Neck and shoulder tension

The good news is that simple TMJ exercises can help improve mobility, reduce discomfort, and restore full function over time.

TMJ Exercises to Improve Jaw Mobility and Strength

1. Controlled Mouth Opening (Stretching Exercise)

Purpose: Improves jaw flexibility and increases range of motion.

How to do it:

1. Place your tongue on the roof of your mouth.
2. Slowly open your mouth as wide as possible without pain.
3. Hold for 5-10 seconds, then close.
4. Repeat 10 times daily.

2. Chin Tucks (Posture Alignment Exercise)

Purpose: Corrects TMJ alignment and relieves jaw tension.

How to do it:

1. Sit or stand with your back straight.
2. Gently tuck your chin toward your neck, like you're making a double chin.
3. Hold for 5 seconds, then release.
4. Repeat 10 times, maintaining proper posture.

3. Resisted Jaw Opening (Strengthening Exercise)

Purpose: Strengthens TMJ muscles and improves stability.

How to do it:

1. Place your thumb under your chin for resistance.
2. Slowly open your mouth while pressing lightly against your chin.
3. Hold for 5 seconds, then slowly close.
4. Repeat 10 times for muscle activation.

4. Side-to-Side Jaw Movement (Mobility Exercise)

Purpose: Enhances jaw flexibility and reduces stiffness.

How to do it:

1. Place a small pencil or tongue depressor between your teeth.
2. Gently move your jaw side to side while keeping the object in place.
3. Hold for 5 seconds on each side, then return to center.
4. Repeat 10 times to improve jaw coordination.

5. Relaxing Jaw Massage

Purpose: Releases tension and improves blood circulation.

How to do it:

1. Use your fingertips to massage the muscles around your TMJ (near your ears).
2. Apply gentle circular motions for 1-2 minutes on each side.
3. Repeat twice daily, especially before bed.

Keep Your TMJ Healthy

If your Four-Finger Test revealed restricted jaw movement, don't worry! With consistent practice of these TMJ exercises, you can restore mobility, reduce tension, and strengthen your jaw over time.

FACIAL MASSAGES & LYMPHATIC DRAINAGE TECHNIQUES FOR A SCULPTED FACE

Facial massage and lymphatic drainage techniques play a crucial role in detoxifying the skin, reducing puffiness, sculpting facial contours, and promoting a youthful glow. These techniques help in stimulating blood circulation, improving lymphatic flow, and relaxing facial muscles, which can enhance the results of Face Yoga.

Here's a comprehensive guide to various facial massages and lymphatic drainage techniques for a healthy, toned, and sculpted face.

1. The Classic Upward Massage (For Anti-Aging & Firming)

How to Perform:

1. Apply a few drops of facial oil or moisturizer for smooth gliding.
2. Use your palms and fingertips to gently massage the face in upward strokes.
3. Move from the jawline to the cheeks, then up to the forehead.
4. Repeat for 2-3 minutes daily.

Benefits:

- Lifts and firms the skin naturally
- Prevents sagging by counteracting gravity
- Stimulates collagen production for youthful skin

2. The Pinching Massage (For Increased Blood Circulation & Glow)

How to Perform:

1. Use your thumb and index finger to gently pinch the skin along the jawline, cheeks, and forehead.
2. Perform light, rhythmic pinching motions, avoiding excessive pressure.
3. Repeat for 1-2 minutes.

Benefits:

- Boosts blood circulation, giving an instant glow
- Stimulates collagen and elastin production
- Improves skin elasticity and tightens loose skin

3. The Knuckle Massage (For Sculpting & Facial Contouring)

How to Perform:

1. Form a loose fist with both hands.
2. Use your knuckles to massage from the chin to the ears, then from the cheeks to the temples.
3. Move in gentle, upward rolling motions.
4. Repeat for 2-3 minutes.

Benefits:

- Defines and sculpts facial contours
- Enhances jawline sharpness and cheekbone prominence
- Improves lymphatic drainage and reduces puffiness

4. The Temple & Forehead Massage (For Stress Relief & Wrinkle Reduction)

How to Perform:

1. Place your fingertips on your temples and massage in small circular motions.
2. Move toward the center of the forehead in an upward direction.
3. Repeat for 2 minutes.

Benefits:

- Relieves tension headaches and forehead wrinkles
- Promotes relaxation and reduces stress
- Enhances blood circulation in the upper face

5. The Eye Drainage Massage (For Reducing Eye Puffiness & Dark Circles)

How to Perform:

1. Use your ring fingers (they apply the least pressure) to gently tap along the under-eye area.
2. Move in a semi-circle motion from the inner to the outer corners of the eyes.
3. Repeat for 30-60 seconds.

Benefits:

- Reduces under-eye puffiness and dark circles
- Stimulates lymphatic drainage in the delicate eye area
- Relaxes eye strain and refreshes tired eyes

6. The Jawline & Chin Massage (For Slimming & Defining the Lower Face)

How to Perform:

1. Use your index and middle fingers to massage along the jawline in upward strokes.
2. Apply gentle pressure and move from chin to ears.
3. Repeat for 1-2 minutes.

Benefits:

- Helps reduce double chin and sagging skin
- Improves jawline definition and tightens muscles
- Prevents jowl formation and enhances contouring

7. The Lymphatic Drainage Massage (For Detoxifying & De-Puffing the Face)

The lymphatic system is responsible for removing toxins and excess fluid from the body. Stimulating lymphatic drainage can help eliminate puffiness, reduce bloating, and improve skin clarity.

How to Perform:

1. Start at the center of your face and use gentle, outward strokes towards the lymph nodes (near the ears and collarbone).
2. Use your fingertips or gua sha tool to sweep down the sides of your neck to encourage drainage.
3. Perform for 2-3 minutes in the morning and evening.

Benefits:

- Reduces facial bloating and puffiness
- Detoxifies and brightens the skin
- Enhances circulation and natural glow

8. The Tapping Massage (For Revitalization & Energy Boost)

How to Perform:

1. Use your fingertips to gently tap all over your face, starting from the forehead to the jawline.
2. Continue for 1-2 minutes using light, rhythmic tapping.

Benefits:

- Boosts oxygen supply to the skin
- Increases energy flow and skin vitality
- Enhances product absorption

9. The Neck & Décolletage Massage (For Preventing Wrinkles & Lifting the Neck Area)

How to Perform:

1. Use your palms to gently stroke upward from the collarbone to the jawline.
2. Apply light pressure and repeat for 2 minutes.
3. Finish by massaging in circular motions at the base of the neck.

Benefits:

- Prevents neck wrinkles and sagging
- Tightens and lifts the neck muscles
- Improves lymphatic drainage for a youthful look

10. The Gua Sha & Facial Roller Technique (For Deep Sculpting & Relaxation)

How to Perform:

1. Apply a light facial oil or serum.
2. Using a gua sha tool or jade roller, glide along the jawline, cheeks, and forehead in upward motions.
3. Use the smaller end of the tool for the under-eye and brow areas.
4. Repeat for 3-5 minutes.

Benefits:

- Lifts and sculpts facial features
- Reduces puffiness and boosts circulation
- Relieves muscle tension and enhances relaxation

Precautions While Performing Facial Massage & Lymphatic Drainage

- Always use gentle pressure to avoid excessive pulling on the skin.
- Use hydrating serums or oils to prevent friction.
- Perform in upward motions to counteract gravity.
- Be consistent but avoid over-massaging (2-3 minutes is sufficient).
- Stay hydrated to maximise lymphatic drainage benefits.

Conclusion

Facial massages and lymphatic drainage techniques enhance the benefits of Face Yoga by promoting detoxification, reducing puffiness, and sculpting facial contours. Regular practice of these techniques will help maintain firm, glowing, and youthful-looking skin—naturally!

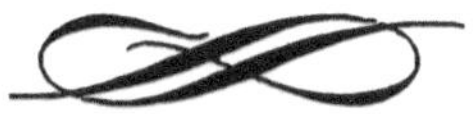

PRECAUTIONS TO TAKE WHILE PRACTICING FACE YOGA

Face Yoga is a natural and effective way to tone facial muscles, improve circulation, and enhance skin elasticity. However, like any exercise, it should be performed correctly and mindfully to avoid unwanted side effects such as wrinkles, muscle strain, or tension. Here are some key precautions to follow while practicing Face Yoga:

1. Start with Clean Hands and a Clean Face

Before touching your face, ensure your hands are clean to prevent breakouts, infections, or irritation. Remove any makeup, dirt, or oils to allow your skin to breathe freely during the exercises.

- Tip: Use a gentle cleanser and pat your face dry before starting.

2. Apply a Light Facial Oil or Moisturizer

Performing Face Yoga on dry skin can cause unnecessary friction, leading to fine lines and irritation. Applying a lightweight facial oil or moisturizer ensures smooth movements and added hydration.

- Tip: Use natural oils like rosehip, jojoba, or almond oil to nourish the skin while exercising.

3. Maintain a Light, Gentle Touch

Excessive pressure or pulling on the skin can cause wrinkles, sagging, or overstretched skin over time. The goal is to work the muscles beneath the skin, not stretch the skin itself.

- Avoid: Tugging, pinching, or pulling the skin too hard.
- Do: Use light fingertips and upward lifting movements.

4. Keep Your Posture Straight

Your posture plays a significant role in the effectiveness of Face Yoga. A slouched position can create unnecessary tension in the neck and jaw, reducing the benefits of the exercises.

- Tip: Sit or stand with a straight spine, relaxed shoulders, and an open chest for maximum effectiveness.

5. Breathe Deeply and Stay Relaxed

Holding your breath or tensing up can create facial tension and stress, which defeats the purpose of Face Yoga. Always practice deep, mindful breathing to oxygenate the muscles and promote relaxation.

- Tip: Inhale deeply through the nose, hold for a moment, and exhale slowly through the mouth.

6. Avoid Over-Exaggerated Movements

While expressions are important in Face Yoga, overdoing them can create unwanted expression lines and wrinkles. Keep your movements controlled, smooth, and precise rather than overly dramatic.

- Avoid: Raising eyebrows too high, frowning, or excessively pursing lips.
- Do: Focus on gentle yet effective engagement of muscles.

7. Don't Overwork Facial Muscles

Just like body muscles, facial muscles need rest to recover and strengthen. Over-exercising can lead to muscle fatigue, soreness, or even premature wrinkles.

- Tip: Practice Face Yoga 5-6 times a week, allowing a day for rest and recovery.

8. Be Mindful of Existing Skin Conditions

If you have sensitive skin, acne, rosacea, or any skin condition, aggressive facial movements may worsen irritation or inflammation.

- Avoid: Rubbing or pressing on inflamed or sensitive areas.
- Do: Use light pressure and slow movements to avoid aggravation.

9. Stay Hydrated for Maximum Results

Dehydrated skin is more prone to wrinkles and dullness, which can reduce the effectiveness of Face Yoga. Drinking enough water helps flush out toxins and maintain skin elasticity.

- Tip: Drink at least 8 glasses of water daily for glowing, healthy skin.

10. Perform Face Yoga in Front of a Mirror (Initially)

A mirror helps you monitor your movements and expressions to ensure you're doing the exercises correctly. This prevents unintentional tension or incorrect technique.

- Tip: Once confident, you can practice Face Yoga without a mirror, but checking occasionally helps maintain proper form.

11. Avoid Face Yoga If You've Had Recent Facial Procedures

If you've had Botox, fillers, facial surgery, or other cosmetic treatments, Face Yoga might interfere with results or cause complications. Always consult your doctor before starting.

- Tip: Wait at least 4-6 weeks after cosmetic treatments before resuming Face Yoga.

12. Don't Expect Instant Results—Be Patient!

Face Yoga requires consistent practice over time to see noticeable changes. Just like body workouts, results depend on regular effort, lifestyle, and overall skincare habits.

- Tip: Stay consistent and practice for at least 8-12 weeks to see visible improvements.

Conclusion

Face Yoga is a powerful, non-invasive way to lift, tone, and sculpt your face naturally. However, it should be practiced with care, patience, and proper technique to maximize benefits while preventing any negative effects.

BREATH-WORK & MINDFULNESS PRACTICES FOR FACE YOGA

Face Yoga isn't just about exercises and massages—it's a holistic practice that combines breathwork, mindfulness, and relaxation to enhance overall skin health, muscle tone, and emotional well-being. Breathwork improves oxygen circulation, reduces stress-induced wrinkles, and enhances lymphatic drainage, while mindfulness helps you connect deeply with your facial muscles and energy.

Here's a comprehensive guide to integrating breathwork and mindfulness practices into your Face Yoga routine for radiant, youthful skin.

1. Diaphragmatic Breathing (Deep Belly Breathing for Relaxation & Glow)

How to Perform:

1. Sit or lie down comfortably, keeping your back straight.
2. Place one hand on your chest and the other on your belly.
3. Inhale deeply through your nose, allowing your belly to expand (not your chest).
4. Exhale slowly through your mouth, feeling your belly contract.
5. Repeat for 5 minutes before starting Face Yoga.

Benefits:

- Reduces stress and tension in facial muscles
- Improves oxygen supply to skin cells for a natural glow
- Enhances lymphatic flow to reduce puffiness

2. Alternate Nostril Breathing (For Facial Symmetry & Balance)

Also known as "Nadi Shodhana," this technique helps balance the nervous system, oxygenate the skin, and promote facial symmetry.

How to Perform:

1. Sit comfortably and close your eyes.
2. Use your right thumb to close your right nostril and inhale deeply through the left nostril.
3. Close your left nostril with your ring finger, release the right nostril, and exhale.
4. Inhale through the right nostril, close it, release the left nostril, and exhale.
5. Continue alternating for 5 minutes.

Benefits:

- Promotes facial balance and symmetry
- Relaxes facial muscles, reducing wrinkles and tension
- Enhances skin detoxification through better oxygenation

3. Lion's Breath (For a Tension-Free, Wrinkle-Free Face)

How to Perform:

1. Sit comfortably and take a deep inhale through your nose.
2. Open your mouth wide, stick your tongue out, and exhale forcefully while making a "ha" sound.
3. Repeat 5 times.

Benefits:

- Releases tension from the jaw, neck, and forehead
- Prevents expression lines and deep wrinkles
- Strengthens facial muscles and improves circulation

4. Humming Bee Breath (Bhramari for Relaxing the Face & Mind)

How to Perform:

1. Close your eyes and take a deep breath in through your nose.
2. As you exhale, make a gentle humming sound like a bee (mmmm).
3. Focus on the vibration in your cheeks, lips, and forehead.
4. Repeat for 5-10 rounds.

Benefits:

- Stimulates facial nerves for a youthful glow
- Reduces stress-related tension in the face
- Improves blood circulation for brighter skin

5. Mindful Face Scanning (For Awareness & Relaxation)

How to Perform:

1. Close your eyes and take three deep breaths.
2. Bring your attention to your forehead—notice any tension and consciously relax it.
3. Move to your eyes, cheeks, lips, jaw, and neck, softening each area with awareness.
4. End by visualizing your entire face glowing and tension-free.

Benefits:

- Enhances mind-muscle connection for better Face Yoga results
- Prevents unconscious facial tension and expression lines
- Promotes deep relaxation for youthful, stress-free skin

6. 4-7-8 Breathing (For Better Oxygen Flow & Skin Rejuvenation)

How to Perform:

1. Inhale deeply through your nose for 4 seconds.
2. Hold your breath for 7 seconds.
3. Exhale slowly through your mouth for 8 seconds.
4. Repeat 5 times before your Face Yoga routine.

Benefits:

- Increases oxygen supply to the skin, reducing dullness
- Calms the nervous system, preventing stress-induced wrinkles
- Boosts lymphatic drainage, reducing puffiness

7. Gratitude & Self-Love Affirmations (For a Positive, Youthful Glow)

Your mindset directly affects how you look and feel. Adding affirmations to your Face Yoga practice enhances its effects.

How to Perform:

1. While practicing Face Yoga, repeat positive affirmations like:

- "My face is lifted, toned, and radiant."
- "I release all tension and welcome relaxation."
- "Every day, my skin glows with youth and vitality."

2. Say them out loud or in your mind with intention.

Benefits:

- Promotes self-confidence and self-love
- Reduces stress and enhances facial relaxation
- Creates a positive mind-body connection for beauty

How to Incorporate Breathwork & Mindfulness into Face Yoga

- Start every session with a breathing exercise to relax and oxygenate your skin.
- Combine breathwork with Face Yoga—exhale during movements to enhance relaxation.
- Practice mindfulness by focusing on each movement and the muscles being engaged.
- End with gratitude affirmations for a self-love boost and glowing skin.

Conclusion

Integrating breathwork and mindfulness into Face Yoga enhances circulation, detoxification, and relaxation, leading to firmer, glowing, and youthful skin. By combining movement, breath, and awareness, you not only transform your face but also cultivate a deep sense of inner peace and well-being.

Breathe, lift, and glow!

TIMELESS BEAUTY: NATURAL SECRETS TO AGING GRACEFULLY

Aging is a natural process, but with the right lifestyle choices, you can slow down its effects and maintain youthful, glowing skin. While there is no way to completely stop aging, natural remedies and lifestyle adjustments can help reduce wrinkles, fine lines, and other signs of aging without relying on expensive treatments or invasive procedures.

This guide covers effective, natural anti-aging hacks that support skin health, boost collagen production, and promote overall well-being.

1. Follow a Skin-Nourishing Diet

Your diet plays a crucial role in skin health and aging. Eating the right foods can enhance collagen production, improve elasticity, and prevent premature aging.

   a.   Best Anti-Aging Foods

- Avocados – Rich in healthy fats, vitamin E, and antioxidants that keep skin hydrated.
- Berries (Blueberries, Strawberries, Raspberries) – Packed with antioxidants that fight free radicals.
- Nuts & Seeds (Almonds, Walnuts, Flaxseeds, Chia Seeds) – Contain omega-3 fatty acids and vitamin E to improve skin elasticity.

- Leafy Greens (Spinach, Kale) – Provide vitamins A, C, and K to boost collagen and reduce wrinkles.
- Fatty Fish (Salmon, Mackerel, Sardines) – High in omega-3s, which help keep skin supple and reduce inflammation.
- Tomatoes – Contain lycopene, which protects against sun damage.
- Green Tea – Loaded with polyphenols that slow down aging and reduce skin inflammation.
- Dark Chocolate (70% cocoa or more) – Contains flavonoids that enhance skin hydration and elasticity.

b. Foods to Avoid

- Processed Sugars & High-Glycemic Foods – Cause glycation, which breaks down collagen and accelerates aging.
- Fried & Fast Foods – Increase inflammation and lead to dull, wrinkled skin.
- Excessive Alcohol & Caffeine – Dehydrates the skin, making fine lines more visible.
- Artificial Trans Fats & Hydrogenated Oils – Damage cell membranes and promote aging.

2. Stay Hydrated

Drinking enough water is one of the simplest and most effective anti-aging habits.

Benefits of Proper Hydration:

- Keeps skin plump and reduces the appearance of wrinkles.
- Helps flush out toxins, preventing acne and dull skin.
- Maintains skin elasticity and promotes a healthy glow.

Tip: Aim for 8-10 glasses of water per day, and add lemon, cucumber, or mint for extra hydration and detox benefits.

3. Get Quality Sleep

Poor sleep accelerates aging and causes dark circles, sagging skin, and dullness.

Natural Sleep Hacks for Anti-Aging

- Stick to a Sleep Schedule – Aim for 7-9 hours of sleep per night.
- Use Silk or Satin Pillowcases – Reduces friction, preventing wrinkles and hair breakage.
- Sleep on Your Back – Prevents "sleep lines" on your face.
- Limit Blue Light Exposure – Avoid screens 1-2 hours before bedtime to boost melatonin production.

4. Protect Your Skin from Sun Damage

UV rays are the biggest cause of premature aging. Too much sun exposure leads to wrinkles, sunspots, and collagen breakdown.

Natural Sun Protection Hacks

- Wear Natural Sunscreen – Use zinc oxide or titanium dioxide-based sunscreens (SPF 30+).
- Use Antioxidant-Rich Oils – Raspberry seed oil and carrot seed oil provide natural sun protection.
- Wear Sunglasses & Hats – Protect delicate facial skin from UV rays.
- Avoid Peak Sun Hours – Stay in the shade between 10 AM - 4 PM.

5. Follow a Consistent Skincare Routine

A simple yet effective skincare routine is key to maintaining healthy, clear, and youthful skin. Follow this basic daily routine:

Morning Routine

- Cleanser – Removes overnight oil and dirt buildup.
- Toner – Balances pH and preps skin for absorption.

- Serum – Apply Vitamin C or Hyaluronic Acid for hydration and brightness.
- Moisturizer – Hydrates and locks in moisture.
- Sunscreen (SPF 30-50) – Protects against premature aging and sun damage.

Night Routine (To Repair & Nourish)

- Double Cleanse – First with an oil-based cleanser, then a gentle face wash.
- Exfoliation (2-3 times a week) – Removes dead skin cells for better product absorption.
- Serum & Treatment – Use retinol, peptides, or niacinamide for anti-aging benefits.
- Moisturizer/Night Cream – Keeps skin hydrated overnight.
- Facial Oil (Optional) – Locks in moisture and promotes overnight repair.

6. Use Natural Oils for Youthful Skin

Natural oils nourish the skin, prevent wrinkles, and enhance elasticity.

Best Anti-Aging Oils

- Argan Oil – Rich in antioxidants and fatty acids to hydrate skin.
- Rosehip Oil – High in vitamin C, promotes collagen production.
- Jojoba Oil – Mimics natural skin oils, keeping skin balanced.
- Coconut Oil – Moisturizes and protects against dryness.
- Almond Oil – Contains vitamin E to repair skin damage.

How to Use: Apply a few drops before bed as a night serum.

7. Facial Exercises & Massage

Facial exercises (also known as "face yoga") help tone the muscles, improve blood circulation, and reduce sagging.

Facial Massage Benefits

- Stimulates collagen production.
- Improves lymphatic drainage to reduce puffiness.
- Relieves tension that leads to wrinkles.

8. Manage Stress Naturally

Chronic stress leads to cortisol spikes, which break down collagen and cause premature aging.

Natural Stress-Reduction Techniques

- Meditation & Deep Breathing – Lowers stress and improves skin health.
- Yoga & Exercise – Boosts circulation and collagen production.
- Aromatherapy – Lavender and chamomile oils promote relaxation.

9. Avoid Smoking & Limit Alcohol

- Smoking reduces oxygen supply to skin, causing wrinkles and dullness.
- Alcohol dehydrates skin and reduces vitamin absorption.

Tip: Swap alcohol for antioxidant-rich drinks like herbal teas, fresh fruit juices, or coconut water.

10. Boost Collagen Naturally

Collagen keeps skin firm and youthful, but declines with age. Increase collagen production naturally with:

a. Collagen-Boosting Foods

- Bone broth
- Egg whites
- Berries
- Citrus fruits (oranges, lemons)
- Garlic

b. Supplements

- Vitamin C – Essential for collagen synthesis.
- Zinc – Helps repair skin.
- Silica – Supports collagen formation.

Final Thoughts

Aging gracefully doesn't require expensive treatments. By following a holistic approach—focusing on diet, hydration, skincare, sleep, and stress management—you can slow down aging naturally and maintain a youthful, radiant complexion.

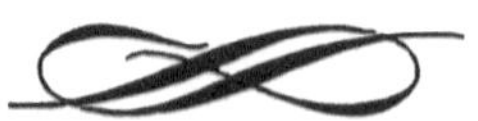

THIRSTY SKIN? SIMPLE AT-HOME TESTS FOR DEHYDRATION

Skin dehydration is a common issue that can lead to dullness, tightness, increased sensitivity, and premature aging. Unlike dry skin, which is a skin type lacking oil, dehydrated skin is a condition that occurs when the skin lacks water. Even people with oily or combination skin can experience dehydration. If your skin feels tight, looks dull, or you notice fine lines appearing more pronounced, your skin might be dehydrated. The good news? You can perform simple at-home tests to check for dehydration and take steps to restore your skin's moisture balance.

1. The Pinch Test (Elasticity Test)

This is the most common test to quickly check if your skin lacks hydration.

How to Perform the Pinch Test:

1. Choose a small area of skin, preferably on your cheek or back of your hand.
2. Gently pinch the skin and hold for a few seconds.
3. Release and observe how quickly the skin returns to normal.

Results:

- If the skin bounces back immediately, your skin is well-hydrated.
- If the skin takes a few seconds to return to normal, your skin is likely dehydrated.

Why does this happen? Hydrated skin is plump and elastic, while dehydrated skin loses its flexibility, making it slower to return to its natural state.

2. The Forehead Shine Test

Dehydrated skin often compensates by producing excess oil, making your forehead appear shiny yet tight or flaky at the same time.

How to Perform the Forehead Test:

1. Wash your face with a gentle cleanser and don't apply any moisturizer.
2. Wait 30 minutes to an hour.
3. Stand in front of a mirror under natural light and observe your forehead.

Results:

- If your forehead looks hydrated but not overly shiny, your skin is balanced.
- If your forehead is shiny but still feels dry or tight, your skin may be overproducing oil to compensate for dehydration.

3. The Lip Test

Dehydration doesn't just affect your facial skin—it also impacts your lips.

How to Perform the Lip Test:

1. Look at your lips closely in the mirror.
2. Lightly press your lips together and notice how they feel.

Results:

- Soft, smooth lips mean your skin is well-hydrated.
- If your lips are cracked, flaky, or feel tight, you may be dehydrated.

4. The Under-Eye Crease Test

One of the first areas to show dehydration is the under-eye area, where skin is thinner and more delicate.

How to Perform the Under-Eye Test:

1.   Look at your under-eye area in natural lighting.
2.   Lightly pull the skin downward and observe for fine lines and creases.

Results:

- If the skin remains smooth, your hydration levels are good.
- If fine lines or creases become more visible when you pull the skin down, your under-eye area is dehydrated.

5. The Makeup Absorption Test

If your skin is dehydrated, foundation and concealer may cling to dry patches or settle into fine lines.

How to Perform the Makeup Test:

1.   Apply your usual foundation or concealer.
2.   Check how it sits on your skin after 30 minutes.

Results:

- If your makeup looks even and smooth, your skin is well-hydrated.
- If your makeup settles into fine lines, looks patchy, or clings to dry areas, your skin is dehydrated.

How to Rehydrate Your Skin at Home

If your skin fails any of these tests, don't worry! You can restore hydration by following these simple steps:

1. Increase Water Intake

- Drink at least 8 glasses of water daily.
- Add hydrating foods like watermelon, cucumber, and oranges to your diet.

2. Use a Hydrating Skincare Routine

- Choose a gentle, non-stripping cleanser.
- Use hydrating serums with hyaluronic acid or glycerin.
- Apply a lightweight but nourishing moisturizer to lock in hydration.

3. Avoid Dehydrating Skincare Habits

- Limit alcohol and caffeine (both dehydrate your skin).
- Avoid over-washing or using harsh cleansers.
- Don't skip moisturizer, even if you have oily skin.

4. Use a Humidifier

- If you live in a dry climate or use air conditioning/heating, a humidifier can restore moisture in the air, preventing your skin from drying out.

5. Hydrating Face Masks

- Try DIY hydration masks with ingredients like honey, aloe vera, and yogurt to restore skin moisture.

KNOWING YOUR SKIN TYPE CHOOSING THE RIGHT SKIN CARE ROUTINE

Understanding your skin type is the foundation of a good skincare routine. If you don't know whether your skin is oily, dry, combination, sensitive, or normal, you might be using the wrong products—leading to breakouts, irritation, or ineffective results.

Luckily, you don't need a dermatologist to determine your skin type. There are simple at-home tests that can help you figure out what your skin needs. Once you identify your skin type, you can choose the right products and build a skincare routine that works for you.

At-Home Skin Type Tests

1. The Bare-Face Test

This is the easiest way to determine your skin type without any special tools.

How to Do It:

1. Wash your face with a gentle cleanser.
2. Do not apply any moisturizer, serum, or toner.
3. Wait for 30 minutes to an hour.
4. Observe how your skin feels and looks.

Results:

- Oily Skin → Your skin looks shiny and greasy, especially in the T-zone.

- Dry Skin → Your skin feels tight, rough, or flaky.
- Combination Skin → Your T-zone is oily, but your cheeks are dry or normal.
- Normal Skin → Your skin feels comfortable and balanced.
- Sensitive Skin → Your skin may appear red, irritated, or slightly itchy.

2. The Blotting Sheet Test

This test helps determine how much oil your skin produces.

How to Do It:

1. Wash your face and pat dry (do not apply moisturizer).
2. Wait for 30-60 minutes.
3. Press an oil blotting sheet or tissue paper on different areas of your face (forehead, nose, cheeks, and chin).
4. Hold the blotting paper up to the light and check for oil.

Results:

- Oily Skin → The blotting sheet absorbs a lot of oil from all areas.
- Dry Skin → The blotting sheet picks up little to no oil.
- Combination Skin → The blotting sheet absorbs oil from the T-zone but not from the cheeks.
- Normal Skin → The blotting sheet absorbs minimal oil but not excessive amounts.
- Sensitive Skin → This test may cause slight redness or irritation if your skin is sensitive.

3. The Pore Size Test

Your pore size can also reveal your skin type.

How to Do It:

1. Stand in front of a mirror under good lighting.
2. Look closely at the pores on your nose, cheeks, and forehead.

Results:

- Oily Skin → Large, visible pores, especially in the T-zone.
- Dry Skin → Very small, barely visible pores.
- Combination Skin → Large pores in the T-zone but smaller pores on the cheeks.
- Normal Skin → Medium-sized pores that are not too visible.
- Sensitive Skin → Pores may appear normal but can be red or inflamed from irritation.

What to Do After Identifying Your Skin Type

Now that you know your skin type, you can choose the right skincare routine:

For Oily Skin

- Use gel-based or foaming cleansers.
- Apply oil-free, lightweight moisturizers.
- Use salicylic acid or niacinamide for oil control.
- Exfoliate 2-3 times a week to prevent clogged pores.

For Dry Skin

- Use a hydrating cream cleanser.
- Apply rich, nourishing moisturizers.
- Use hyaluronic acid, ceramides, and glycerin for deep hydration.
- Avoid alcohol-based toners and harsh exfoliants.

For Combination Skin

- Use a gentle, balancing cleanser.
- Apply a light moisturizer on oily areas and a heavier one on dry areas.
- Use clay masks for the T-zone and hydrating masks for dry cheeks.

For Normal Skin

- Use a mild cleanser and lightweight moisturizer.
- Stick to a simple, balanced skincare routine.
- Maintain hydration and sun protection.

For Sensitive Skin

- Choose fragrance-free, gentle products.
- Use soothing ingredients like aloe vera and chamomile.
- Avoid harsh exfoliants and alcohol-based toners.
- Always patch-test new products before applying them.

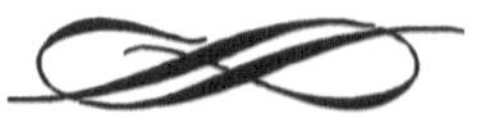

DEW IT RIGHT: A SMART GUIDE TO CHOOSING MOISTURIZERS

Moisturizing is a key step in any skincare routine, helping to maintain hydration, protect the skin barrier, and address specific skin concerns. However, with countless options available, selecting the right moisturizer can feel overwhelming. This guide will help you understand the different types of moisturizers, essential ingredients, and how to choose the best one based on your skin type and needs.

Moisturizers come in different formulations to suit various skin needs. Here are the primary types:

a. Humectants

  - Attract water from the environment into the skin.
  - Best for dehydrated or dry skin.
  - Common ingredients: Hyaluronic Acid, Glycerin, Aloe Vera.

b. Emollients

  - Smooth and soften the skin by filling in cracks between skin cells.
  - Ideal for normal to dry skin.
  - Common ingredients: Shea Butter, Squalane, Ceramides.

c. Occlusives

  - Create a barrier to lock in moisture and prevent water loss.
  - Best for extremely dry or damaged skin.
  - Common ingredients: Petroleum Jelly, Beeswax, Mineral Oil.

d. Gel-Based Moisturizers

- Lightweight and water-based.
- Perfect for oily, acne-prone, or combination skin.
- Absorbs quickly without leaving a greasy residue.

e. Cream-Based Moisturizers

- Thicker and richer in consistency.
- Suitable for dry and sensitive skin.
- Provides deep hydration and nourishment.

f. Lotion-Based Moisturizers

- Lighter than creams but more hydrating than gels.
- Good for normal to combination skin.

g. Oil-Based Moisturizers

- Contain plant-based or essential oils for extra nourishment.
- Best for dry or mature skin.

Choosing the Right Moisturizer for Your Skin Type

Here's a breakdown of which moisturizer suits each skin type:

a. Best Moisturizer for Normal Skin

- Choose lightweight lotions that maintain balance.
- Look for hydrating but non-greasy formulas.
- Key Ingredients: Hyaluronic Acid, Squalane, Vitamin E.

b. Best Moisturizer for Dry Skin

- Opt for thicker creams or oil-based moisturizers.
- Look for occlusive ingredients to lock in moisture.
- Key Ingredients: Shea Butter, Ceramides, Glycerin, Squalane.

c. Best Moisturizer for Oily Skin

- Go for oil-free, non-comedogenic, gel-based formulas.
- Look for ingredients that control oil while keeping the skin hydrated.
- Key Ingredients: Hyaluronic Acid, Niacinamide, Aloe Vera.

d. Best Moisturizer for Combination Skin

- Use a lightweight lotion or gel-based moisturizer.
- Avoid heavy creams in oily areas.
- Key Ingredients: Hyaluronic Acid, Glycerin, Aloe Vera.

e. Best Moisturizer for Sensitive Skin

- Choose fragrance-free, hypoallergenic formulas.
- Avoid alcohol, artificial dyes, and harsh chemicals.
- Key Ingredients: Ceramides, Oat Extract, Aloe Vera, Chamomile.

f. Best Moisturizer for Acne-Prone Skin

- Opt for oil-free, lightweight, and non-comedogenic products.
- Look for soothing and acne-fighting ingredients.
- Key Ingredients: Niacinamide, Hyaluronic Acid, Tea Tree Oil, Salicylic Acid.

Key Ingredients to Look for in a Moisturizer

- Hyaluronic Acid – Deeply hydrates without making skin greasy.
- Glycerin – Draws moisture into the skin, keeping it plump.
- Niacinamide (Vitamin B3) – Regulates oil production and soothes inflammation.
- Ceramides – Strengthen the skin barrier and retain moisture.
- Aloe Vera – Soothes irritation and hydrates.
- Squalane – Mimics natural skin oils, keeping skin balanced.

- Shea Butter – Provides rich nourishment and protection.
- Vitamin E – Repairs and protects against environmental damage.

Ingredients to Avoid Based on Skin Type

a. If You Have Oily or Acne-Prone Skin:

   - Heavy Oils (Coconut Oil, Mineral Oil)
   - Alcohol (Denatured Alcohol)
   - Silicones (Dimethicone)
   - Fragrance & Essential Oils

b. If You Have Sensitive Skin:

   - Fragrance & Dyes
   - Alcohol
   - Harsh Acids (High concentration AHAs & BHAs)
   - Parabens & Sulfates

c. If You Have Dry Skin:

   - Foaming agents (like Sodium Lauryl Sulfate, SLS)
   - Oil-free formulas (not enough hydration)

Additional Tips for Choosing a Moisturizer

- Check the Label: Look for "non-comedogenic" for acne-prone skin and "hypoallergenic" for sensitive skin.
- SPF Protection: If using a daytime moisturizer, opt for SPF 30 or higher.
- Patch Test: Always test new products on a small area before full application.
- Seasonal Adjustments: Use lightweight moisturizers in summer and heavier ones in winter.
- Consistency Matters: Stick to a routine for best results.

Final Thoughts

Choosing the right moisturizer is essential for healthy, glowing skin. By understanding your skin type, selecting the appropriate ingredients, and avoiding harmful components, you can maintain balanced, hydrated, and youthful-looking skin. Regularly reassess your skin's needs, adjust your routine based on the seasons, and be consistent for the best results.

GLOW IN A BOTTLE: HOW TO CHOOSE THE RIGHT SERUM

1. Understanding What a Serum Does

A serum is a concentrated skincare product designed to:

- Deliver potent active ingredients deep into the skin
- Target specific concerns like wrinkles, dark spots, acne, and dryness
- Provide faster and more noticeable results than regular moisturizers

   Unlike moisturizers, serums have smaller molecules, allowing them to penetrate the skin more effectively.

2. How to Choose the Right Serum for Your Skin Type & Concern

(A) Serums for Dry & Dehydrated Skin

Look for: Hydrating and moisture-retaining ingredients.

- Hyaluronic Acid – Attracts and locks in moisture for plump skin.
- Glycerin – Prevents moisture loss and keeps skin supple.
- Panthenol (Vitamin B5) – Deeply hydrates and soothes dryness.
- Squalane – Mimics natural skin oils for long-lasting hydration.

Best Serums:

- Hydrating Hyaluronic Acid Serum
- Aloe Vera & Squalane Serum

Pro Tip: Apply on damp skin and follow with a moisturizer to seal in hydration.

(B) Serums for Oily & Acne-Prone Skin

Look for: Lightweight, non-comedogenic ingredients that regulate oil and fight acne.

- Niacinamide (Vitamin B3) – Controls sebum, reduces pores, and brightens skin.
- Salicylic Acid (BHA) – Exfoliates, unclogs pores, and prevents breakouts.
- Tea Tree Oil – Has antibacterial properties to fight acne.
- Zinc – Controls oil production and reduces inflammation.

Best Serums:

- Niacinamide + Zinc Serum
- Salicylic Acid Acne Serum

Pro Tip: Avoid heavy oils and use gel-based or water-based serums.

(C) Serums for Sensitive & Redness-Prone Skin

Look for: Soothing, anti-inflammatory ingredients that calm irritation.

- Centella Asiatica (Cica) – Reduces redness and repairs the skin barrier.
- Chamomile & Green Tea Extract – Calms inflammation and hydrates.
- Aloe Vera – Soothes and reduces sensitivity.
- Beta-Glucan – Strengthens the skin's natural defense system.

Best Serums:

- Centella & Green Tea Serum
- Aloe Vera & Panthenol Serum

Pro Tip: Avoid alcohol, fragrance, and harsh exfoliants.

(D) Serums for Dull & Uneven Skin Tone

Look for: Brightening and exfoliating ingredients.

- Vitamin C – Fades dark spots, boosts collagen, and enhances radiance.
- Alpha Arbutin – Reduces hyperpigmentation and evens skin tone.
- Kojic Acid – Helps lighten dark spots and acne scars.
- Licorice Extract – Brightens skin and reduces sun damage.

Best Serums:

- Vitamin C + Hyaluronic Acid Serum
- Alpha Arbutin + Kojic Acid Serum

Pro Tip: Use Vitamin C in the morning with sunscreen to prevent further pigmentation.

(E) Serums for Aging & Wrinkles (Anti-Aging Serums)

Look for: Ingredients that boost collagen, firm skin, and reduce wrinkles.

- Retinol (Vitamin A) – Increases collagen production and smooths fine lines.
- Peptides – Strengthens skin and boosts elasticity.
- Bakuchiol (Retinol Alternative) – Gentle plant-based anti-aging ingredient.
- Coenzyme Q10 (CoQ10) – Protects skin from environmental damage and aging.

Best Serums:

- Retinol + Peptides Serum
- Bakuchiol + Hyaluronic Acid Serum

Pro Tip: Use retinol at night and always wear sunscreen in the morning.

(F) Serums for Hyperpigmentation & Dark Spots

Look for: Skin-lightening and exfoliating ingredients.

- Vitamin C – Brightens and prevents pigmentation.
- Alpha Arbutin – Reduces dark spots and evens skin tone.
- Azelaic Acid – Treats pigmentation and acne scars.
- Tranexamic Acid – Reduces stubborn melasma and discoloration.

Best Serums:

- Vitamin C + Alpha Arbutin Serum
- Azelaic Acid Brightening Serum

Pro Tip: Always use SPF with brightening serums to prevent further pigmentation.

3. How to Use a Serum Correctly

- Cleanse Your Face – Start with a gentle face wash.
- Apply a Toner – Prepares skin for better absorption.
- Apply 2-3 Drops of Serum – Gently pat into your skin, don't rub.
- Follow with a Moisturizer – Locks in the serum's benefits.
- Use Sunscreen (Daytime Only) – Essential if using Vitamin C or retinol.

Frequency:

- Hydrating serums (Hyaluronic Acid) – Twice daily.
- Vitamin C serums – Morning only.

- Retinol & exfoliating serums (AHA/BHA) – Night only, 2-3 times a week.

4. Common Mistakes to Avoid

- Overusing serums – Too many active ingredients can irritate the skin.
- Mixing incompatible ingredients – Avoid combining retinol with Vitamin C or AHAs/BHAs with Niacinamide.
- Skipping sunscreen – Ingredients like Vitamin C, retinol, and exfoliants make skin sun-sensitive.
- Using too much serum – A few drops are enough; over-application won't enhance results.

5. Choosing a Serum Based on Skin Type

Skin Type	Best Serums
Dry Skin	Hyaluronic Acid, Squalane, Vitamin B5
Oily Skin	Niacinamide, Salicylic Acid, Zinc
Sensitive Skin	Centella Asiatica, Chamomile, Aloe Vera
Dull Skin	Vitamin C, Alpha Arbutin, Kojic Acid
Aging Skin	Retinol, Peptides, CoQ10
Hyperpigmentation	Tranexamic Acid, Azelaic Acid, Licorice

Conclusion

Choosing the right serum depends on your skin type, specific concerns, and skincare goals. Whether you need hydration, anti-aging, brightening, or acne control, the right serum can transform your skin when used correctly.

Pro Tip: Start with one active ingredient at a time, stay consistent, and always protect your skin with moisturizer and sunscreen for the best results.

Glow smart, glow naturally!

FIRM & FABULOUS: HOMEMADE MASKS FOR SKIN TIGHTENING

Aging gracefully doesn't have to be expensive! With natural ingredients rich in antioxidants, vitamins, and skin-tightening properties, you can create powerful DIY anti-aging and skin-firming masks at home. These masks help reduce fine lines, improve elasticity, and give your skin a youthful glow.

1. Egg White & Honey Firming Mask

Why It Works:

- Egg whites tighten and firm the skin.
- Honey hydrates and nourishes, reducing fine lines.

Ingredients:

- 1 egg white
- 1 teaspoon honey
- ½ teaspoon lemon juice (optional, for brightening)

Directions:

1. Whisk the egg white until frothy.
2. Mix in honey and lemon juice.
3. Apply evenly to the face and neck.
4. Leave for 15-20 minutes until it tightens.
5. Rinse with lukewarm water.

Use: 2 times a week.

2. Banana & Yogurt Anti-Wrinkle Mask

Why It Works:

- Banana is rich in vitamins A and C, which reduce wrinkles.
- Yogurt contains lactic acid to gently exfoliate and firm the skin.

Ingredients:

- ½ ripe banana (mashed)
- 1 tablespoon plain yogurt
- 1 teaspoon honey

Directions:

1. Mash the banana until smooth.
2. Mix in yogurt and honey.
3. Apply to your face and leave for 20 minutes.
4. Rinse off with cool water.

Use: 2-3 times a week.

3. Avocado & Olive Oil Hydrating Mask

Why It Works:

- Avocado contains healthy fats that nourish dry, aging skin.
- Olive oil is rich in antioxidants to fight free radicals.

Ingredients:

- ½ ripe avocado (mashed)
- 1 teaspoon olive oil
- 1 teaspoon honey

Directions:

1. Mash the avocado and mix with olive oil and honey.
2. Apply a thick layer to your face and leave for 20 minutes.
3. Wash off with lukewarm water.

Use: 2 times a week.

4. Aloe Vera & Vitamin E Repair Mask

Why It Works:

- Aloe vera boosts collagen production and soothes skin.
- Vitamin E repairs damaged skin and improves elasticity.

Ingredients:

- 2 tablespoons fresh aloe vera gel
- 1 vitamin E capsule (pierce and extract oil)

Directions:

1. Mix aloe vera gel with vitamin E oil.
2. Apply to your face and neck.
3. Leave for 20 minutes, then rinse.

Use: 3 times a week.

5. Cucumber & Rice Flour Tightening Mask

Why It Works:

- Cucumber refreshes and tightens skin.
- Rice flour has anti-aging properties and smoothens skin texture.

Ingredients:

- ½ cucumber (blended)
- 1 tablespoon rice flour
- 1 teaspoon rose water

Directions:

1. Blend the cucumber and mix with rice flour and rose water.
2. Apply to your face and let it dry for 20 minutes.
3. Rinse with cool water.

Use: 2 times a week.

6. Coffee & Cocoa Anti-Aging Mask

Why It Works:

- Coffee contains caffeine, which firms and tightens the skin.
- Cocoa is rich in antioxidants that prevent wrinkles.

Ingredients:

- 1 tablespoon ground coffee
- 1 tablespoon cocoa powder
- 1 tablespoon yogurt or honey

Directions:

1. Mix all ingredients into a paste.
2. Apply and gently massage for 2 minutes.
3. Leave for 15 minutes before rinsing.

Use: 2 times a week.

7. Turmeric & Milk Brightening Mask

Why It Works:

- Turmeric reduces inflammation and evens skin tone.
- Milk contains lactic acid to improve elasticity.

Ingredients:

- 1 teaspoon turmeric powder
- 2 tablespoons milk
- 1 teaspoon honey

Directions:

1. Mix all ingredients well.
2. Apply to the skin and leave for 15 minutes.
3. Wash off with lukewarm water.

Use: 1-2 times a week.

8. Papaya & Honey Anti-Aging Mask

Why It Works:

- Papaya contains natural enzymes that promote skin renewal.
- Honey hydrates and fights free radicals.

Ingredients:

- 2 tablespoons mashed papaya
- 1 teaspoon honey
- ½ teaspoon lemon juice (optional)

Directions:

1. Mix all ingredients into a smooth paste.
2. Apply and leave for 20 minutes.
3. Rinse off with cool water.

Use: 2 times a week.

9. Oatmeal & Almond Anti-Wrinkle Mask

Why It Works:

- Oatmeal soothes and tightens skin.
- Almond powder provides essential nutrients for skin regeneration.

Ingredients:

- 2 tablespoons ground oatmeal
- 1 tablespoon almond powder
- 1 tablespoon yogurt or milk

Directions:

1. Mix ingredients to form a paste.
2. Apply and massage gently for exfoliation.
3. Leave for 15 minutes, then rinse.

Use: 2 times a week.

10. Carrot & Coconut Oil Rejuvenating Mask

Why It Works:

- Carrots are rich in beta-carotene, which boosts collagen.
- Coconut oil deeply hydrates and smooths skin.

Ingredients:

- 1 small carrot (boiled & mashed)
- 1 teaspoon coconut oil
- 1 teaspoon honey

Directions:

1. Mash the cooked carrot and mix with coconut oil and honey.
2. Apply to your face and leave for 20 minutes.
3. Rinse with lukewarm water.

Use: 2 times a week.

Final Tips for Best Results

- Always apply masks to a clean face.
- Use lukewarm water to rinse off masks for better absorption.
- Moisturize after using any mask to lock in hydration.
- Be consistent—natural remedies work best with regular use.
- Patch-test ingredients if you have sensitive skin.

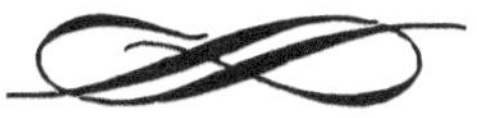

SCRUB IT RIGHT: THE 10 BEST DIY FACE SCRUBS FOR A FRESH GLOW

Exfoliating your skin is key to maintaining a radiant complexion. Store-bought scrubs can be expensive and may contain harsh chemicals, but DIY face scrubs are an easy, natural, and budget-friendly alternative. Here are 10 of the best homemade face scrubs you can make with simple ingredients from your kitchen!

1. Honey & Sugar Scrub (For All Skin Types)

Ingredients:

- 1 tbsp honey
- 1 tbsp granulated sugar (brown or white)

How to Use:

Mix honey and sugar to create a thick paste. Gently massage it onto damp skin for a minute, then rinse with warm water. Honey hydrates while sugar exfoliates.

2. Oatmeal & Yogurt Scrub (For Sensitive Skin)

Ingredients:

- 2 tbsp oatmeal (ground)
- 2 tbsp yogurt
- 1 tsp honey

How to Use:

Mix ingredients into a smooth paste. Apply to your face, gently scrubbing for a minute. Let it sit for a few minutes before rinsing off. This scrub soothes irritation while exfoliating gently.

3. Coffee & Coconut Oil Scrub (For Dull Skin)

Ingredients:

- 1 tbsp coffee grounds
- 1 tbsp coconut oil

How to Use:

Mix and apply in circular motions for about a minute. Rinse with lukewarm water. Coffee stimulates circulation, and coconut oil moisturizes the skin.

4. Baking Soda & Lemon Scrub (For Oily Skin)

Ingredients:

- 1 tbsp baking soda
- ½ tbsp lemon juice
- ½ tbsp honey

How to Use:

Mix ingredients into a paste and gently scrub for 30 seconds. Rinse with cool water. Baking soda removes excess oil, while lemon brightens the skin. Use only once a week to avoid over-exfoliation.

5. Brown Sugar & Olive Oil Scrub (For Dry Skin)

Ingredients:

- 1 tbsp brown sugar
- 1 tbsp olive oil

How to Use:

Mix and rub onto your skin in gentle circular motions. Rinse with warm water. Brown sugar sloughs off dead skin, and olive oil provides deep hydration.

6. Green Tea & Honey Scrub (For Anti-Aging & Detoxifying)

Ingredients:

- 1 tbsp green tea leaves (or a used green tea bag)
- 1 tbsp honey

How to Use:

Mix and gently massage onto the skin. Leave it on for 5 minutes before rinsing. Green tea fights free radicals and reduces inflammation.

7. Sea Salt & Aloe Vera Scrub (For Acne-Prone Skin)

Ingredients:

- 1 tbsp sea salt
- 1 tbsp aloe vera gel

How to Use:

Mix and apply gently to exfoliate without irritating breakouts. Sea salt detoxifies while aloe soothes redness and inflammation.

8. Almond & Milk Scrub (For Brightening & Nourishing Skin)

Ingredients:

- 1 tbsp ground almonds
- 1 tbsp milk

How to Use:

Mix into a paste and apply in circular motions. Leave it on for 5 minutes before rinsing. Almonds exfoliate while milk brightens and nourishes.

9. Strawberry & Sugar Scrub (For Skin Softening & Brightening)

Ingredients:

- 2 mashed strawberries
- 1 tbsp sugar
- ½ tsp honey

How to Use:

Mix and massage onto the skin. Strawberries contain natural AHAs that help brighten and soften skin.

10. Rice Flour & Rose Water Scrub (For Oil Control & Even Skin Tone)

Ingredients:

- 1 tbsp rice flour
- 1 tbsp rose water

How to Use:

Mix into a fine paste and gently exfoliate. Rice flour absorbs excess oil and brightens, while rose water soothes the skin.

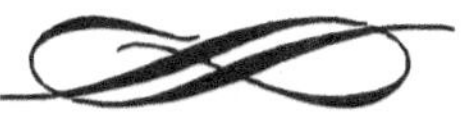

CRYO BEAUTY: HOW ICE CAN TRANSFORM YOUR SKIN

Skin icing is a popular and natural skincare technique that involves applying ice or cold therapy to the skin to achieve a firmer, more radiant, and refreshed complexion. It has been used for centuries in beauty routines to reduce puffiness, tighten pores, and improve circulation.

1. What is Skin Icing?

Skin icing involves using ice cubes, cold compresses, or ice globes to apply cold therapy to the face. It works by constricting blood vessels, reducing inflammation, and improving circulation, which can enhance skin texture and appearance.

Common forms of skin icing include:

- Direct Ice Cube Massage – Applying an ice cube wrapped in a cloth.
- Ice Globes or Cryo Sticks – Special tools designed for facial icing.
- Frozen Cucumber or Green Tea Ice Cubes – Using infused ice for added skincare benefits.
- Cold Water Dunking – Dipping your face in a bowl of ice-cold water.

2. Benefits of Skin Icing

    A. Reduces Puffiness & Under-Eye Bags

- Cold therapy helps constrict blood vessels, reducing swelling and puffiness.
- Great for morning face puffiness or tired eyes.

    B. Tightens Pores & Reduces Oiliness

- Cold temperature shrinks pores and controls excess oil production.
- Helps prevent breakouts and acne by minimizing clogged pores.

    C. Improves Blood Circulation & Enhances Glow

- The shock of cold increases blood flow, bringing oxygen and nutrients to the skin.
- Gives a natural, healthy glow by stimulating skin cells.

    D. Soothes Redness & Irritation

- Helpful for sensitive, sunburned, or inflamed skin.
- Reduces redness from acne, rosacea, or skin irritation.

    E. Helps with Acne & Breakouts

- Reduces inflammation and swelling of active pimples.
- Helps shrink painful cystic acne and prevents further breakouts.

    F. Reduces the Appearance of Fine Lines & Wrinkles

- Temporary skin tightening effect helps reduce fine lines.
- Promotes collagen production over time with regular use.

    G. Enhances Product Absorption

- Using ice before applying serums or moisturizers helps the skin absorb products better.

- Creates a firming and plumping effect when combined with skincare.

3. How to Properly Ice Your Skin

Step-by-Step Guide

- Step 1: Cleanse Your Face – Wash your face to remove dirt and oil.
- Step 2: Wrap Ice in a Soft Cloth – Never apply ice directly to avoid burns.
- Step 3: Gently Massage in Circular Motions – Focus on areas like the cheeks, forehead, under-eyes, and jawline.
- Step 4: Limit to 1-2 Minutes Per Area – Avoid prolonged contact with one spot.
- Step 5: Follow with Serum & Moisturizer – Cold skin absorbs skincare better.

How Often to Ice Your Skin?

- Daily Icing – If your skin tolerates it, 2-3 times a week is ideal.
- Sensitive Skin – Limit to 1-2 times a week to prevent irritation.
- Acne-Prone Skin – Ice individual pimples as needed to reduce swelling.

4. Best Types of Ice Cubes for Skin

Instead of plain water, try infused ice cubes for extra skincare benefits:

- Green Tea Ice Cubes – Rich in antioxidants, reduces acne and inflammation.
- Cucumber Ice Cubes – Soothes, hydrates, and brightens skin.
- Aloe Vera Ice Cubes – Heals sunburn and calms irritation.
- Rose Water Ice Cubes – Refreshes and hydrates dry skin.
- Milk Ice Cubes – Lightens dark spots and provides a smooth glow.

5. Side Effects & Precautions

A. Potential Side Effects of Skin Icing

- Ice Burns & Frostbite – Direct application can damage skin.
- Over-Drying – Excessive icing can strip skin of natural oils.
- Increased Sensitivity – Can worsen redness if you have rosacea.
- Broken Capillaries – Prolonged use can lead to visible veins or sensitivity.

B. Who Should Avoid Skin Icing?

- People with Extremely Dry or Sensitive Skin – Icing may cause irritation.
- Rosacea or Broken Capillaries – Can worsen redness and sensitivity.
- Migraine-Prone Individuals – Sudden cold exposure may trigger headaches.
- Before Makeup Application – Avoid excessive icing, as it can cause patchy makeup application.

C. Best Practices to Avoid Side Effects

- Always wrap ice in a soft cloth – Never apply directly.
- Limit exposure to 1-2 minutes per area – Don't overdo it.
- Follow with hydration – Always apply moisturizer after icing.
- Do a patch test if you have sensitive skin.

6. Alternatives to Ice for a Cooling Effect

If direct ice is too harsh, try gentler cooling methods:

- Chilled Jade Roller or Gua Sha – Provides similar cooling benefits.
- Cold Spoon Therapy – Helps with puffy under-eyes.
- Refrigerated Sheet Masks – A cooling skincare alternative.
- Cold Aloe Vera Gel – Soothes and hydrates skin.

7. Conclusion: Should You Ice Your Skin?

Skin icing is a powerful, natural skincare technique that can enhance radiance, tighten skin, and reduce puffiness. However, it should be done with care to avoid side effects like burns, broken capillaries, and excessive dryness.

When done correctly, icing can be a game-changer for glowing, healthy skin!

Pro Tip: Pair icing with a good skincare routine, hydration, and sun protection for maximum skin benefits.

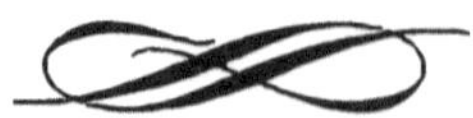

DRENCH & GLOW: THE 100 SPLASHES CLEANSING SECRET

The 100 Splashes Face Wash Method is a traditional skincare technique that involves splashing water on the face 100 times to cleanse, refresh, and invigorate the skin. This technique, rooted in ancient Asian beauty rituals, is known for its hydration, circulation boost, and pore-tightening effects.

1. What is the 100 Splashes Face Wash Method?

The 100 Splashes Wash is a gentle yet effective cleansing method where the face is rinsed with 100 splashes of water after cleansing. It is believed to:

- Deep cleanse without stripping natural oils
- Stimulate blood circulation for a natural glow
- Hydrate and refresh the skin
- Tighten pores and tone the face

This method avoids harsh rubbing or scrubbing, making it suitable for sensitive skin types.

2. Benefits of the 100 Splashes Wash

A. Deeply Hydrates the Skin

- Continuous splashing helps the skin absorb water, preventing dehydration.
- Ideal for dry and dull skin, restoring moisture levels naturally.

B. Improves Blood Circulation & Radiance

- The repetitive motion stimulates microcirculation, delivering oxygen and nutrients.
- Skin looks healthier, fresher, and more radiant.

C. Minimizes Pores & Controls Oil Production

- The cool or lukewarm water tightens pores and regulates sebum.
- Reduces excess oil, preventing clogged pores and acne.

D. Enhances Skin Detoxification

- Helps flush out toxins and pollutants.
- Reduces breakouts and skin congestion.

E. Soothes Irritated Skin

- Reduces redness and calms inflammation.
- Great for sensitive, acne-prone, and combination skin.

F. Provides a Gentle Cleansing Effect

- Ideal for those who want a non-abrasive cleansing method.
- No need for harsh scrubbing or excessive use of products.

3. Step-by-Step Guide to the 100 Splashes Face Wash Method

Step 1: Start with a Gentle Cleanser (Optional)

- If wearing makeup or sunscreen, double cleanse before splashing.
- Use a mild, non-stripping cleanser suitable for your skin type.

Step 2: Prepare Water in a Clean Bowl or Sink

- Use lukewarm or cool water (avoid hot water, as it strips natural oils).
- Optional: Add green tea, rose water, or rice water for added skin benefits.

Step 3: Begin Splashing Your Face

- Using both hands, cup water and splash gently onto your face.
- Splash 100 times, ensuring even distribution.

Step 4: Gently Pat Dry

- Do not rub your skin with a towel; instead, pat dry with a soft, clean towel.

Step 5: Apply Skincare Immediately

- While the skin is damp, apply a hydrating toner, serum, and moisturizer.
- Follow with sunscreen (if done in the morning).

4. Best Practices & Pro Tips

- Use Filtered or Mineral Water – If tap water is harsh, use filtered or cooled boiled water.
- Adjust Water Temperature – Lukewarm water is best; cold water helps with puffiness.
- Be Gentle with Your Skin – No aggressive rubbing or scrubbing.
- Enhance with Natural Ingredients – Add green tea, aloe vera, or rice water for extra benefits.
- Stay Consistent – Try this method 2-3 times a week for visible results.

5. Who Should & Shouldn't Try This Method?

Best for:

- Oily & Combination Skin – Helps regulate excess oil and reduce pores.
- Dull & Tired Skin – Boosts circulation and hydration for a glow.

- Sensitive & Redness-Prone Skin – No harsh scrubbing makes it gentle.
- Aging Skin – Helps with firmness, elasticity, and natural glow.

Avoid If:

- Extremely Dry Skin – Excessive splashing may dehydrate skin further.
- Severe Acne or Open Wounds – Can cause irritation if not done carefully.
- Rosacea or Broken Capillaries – Cold water can worsen redness and sensitivity.

6. Alternatives to the 100 Splashes Method

If 100 splashes feel excessive, try these gentler alternatives:

- 50 Splashes Method – A shorter version that still refreshes the skin.
- Cold Compress – Use a chilled towel for a similar tightening effect.
- Hydrating Face Mist – Spritz water or rose water for hydration.
- Japanese Rice Water Wash – Use fermented rice water for added glow.

7. Conclusion: Is the 100 Splashes Face Wash Worth Trying?

The 100 Splashes Face Wash Method is a simple, natural, and effective technique that can improve hydration, circulation, and skin clarity. When done correctly and consistently, it can be a great addition to your skincare routine.

Pro Tip: Adapt the method to your skin's needs by adjusting the water temperature, splash count, and frequency.

ANTI-AGING HOME TOOLBOX

Using home facial tools can enhance face yoga, massage, and anti-aging exercises by stimulating circulation, collagen production, and muscle toning. This guide covers the most effective tools, their benefits, how to use them correctly, and precautions to maximize results.

1. Gua Sha – Sculpting & Lifting

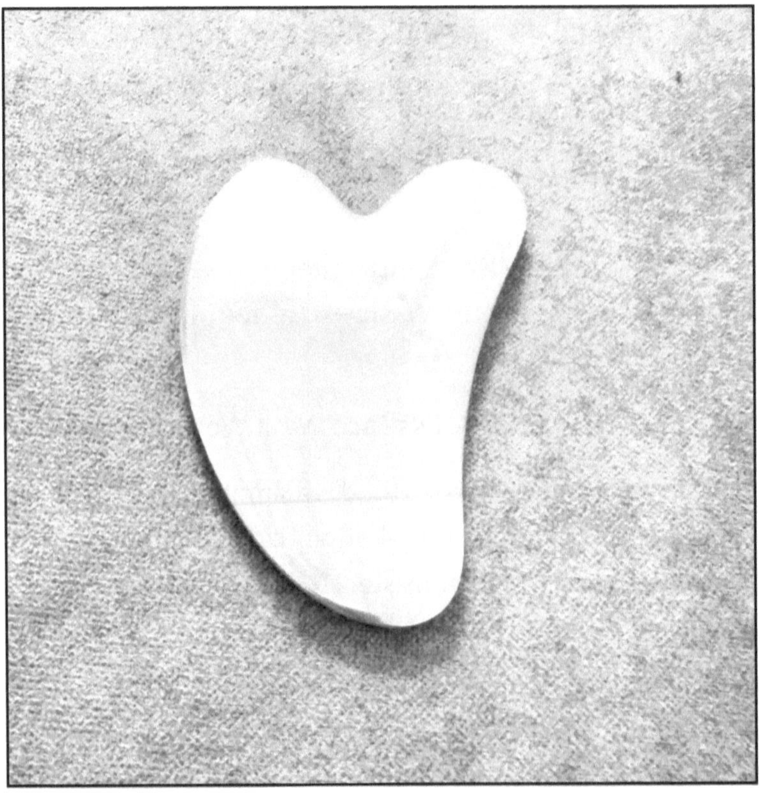

What It Is:

- A flat stone tool (jade, rose quartz, or stainless steel) used for scraping motions on the skin.
- Based on Traditional Chinese Medicine (TCM) to release tension, improve circulation, and contour the face.

Benefits:

- Lifts and sculpts the face
- Boosts lymphatic drainage, reducing puffiness
- Stimulates collagen production
- Relieves jaw tension and improves blood flow

How to Use It:

- Apply a facial oil or serum to prevent friction.
- Hold the gua sha tool flat against the skin.
- Use gentle, upward strokes along the jawline, cheeks, and forehead.
- Use the curved edge for under-eye and brow lifting.
- Repeat for 3–5 minutes daily.

Best For:

- Jawline sculpting, cheek lifting, reducing wrinkles, draining puffiness.

Precautions:

- Avoid aggressive pressure (can cause bruising).
- Don't use on inflamed or irritated skin.

2. Dermaroller – Collagen Boosting & Wrinkle Reduction

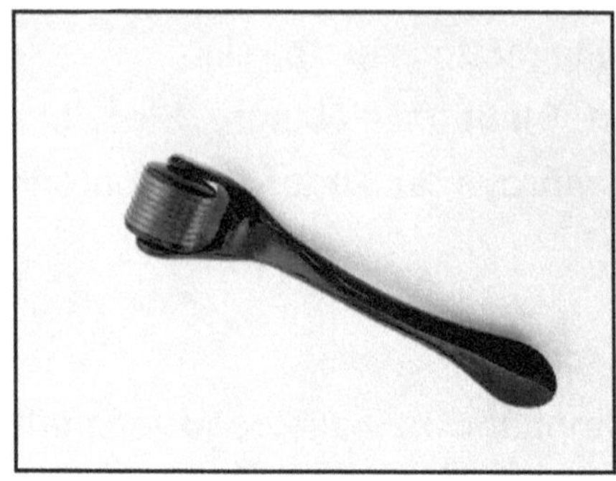

What It Is:

- A roller with micro-needles that creates tiny punctures in the skin to stimulate collagen production and skin renewal.

Benefits:

- Increases collagen & elastin, reducing fine lines
- Enhances product absorption (serums & anti-aging creams)
- Improves skin texture and tightens pores
- Boosts blood circulation for a youthful glow

How to Use It:

- Choose a 0.25mm to 0.5mm needle length for home use.
- Sanitize the roller before and after use.
- Apply a hydrating serum (like hyaluronic acid).
- Gently roll in horizontal, vertical, and diagonal directions across the face.
- Finish with a calming serum or moisturizer.
- Use 1–2 times per week.

Best For:

- Fine lines, wrinkles, sagging skin, acne scars, uneven texture.

Precautions:

- Avoid if you have active acne, sensitive skin, or rosacea.
- Always sanitize before and after use.
- Follow with sunscreen, as skin becomes more sensitive.

3. Jade Roller – Cooling & De-Puffing

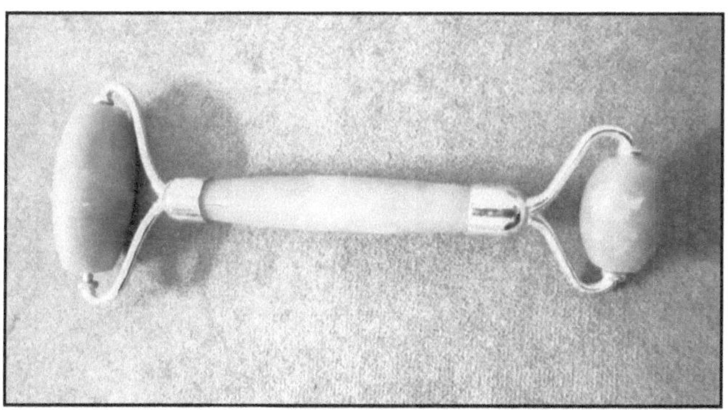

What It Is:

- A smooth jade or rose quartz roller designed for gentle facial massage.

Benefits:

- Reduces puffiness and enhances lymphatic drainage
- Soothes and calms skin
- Increases circulation, giving a natural glow
- Enhances serum absorption

How to Use It:

- Apply a hydrating serum or oil.
- Use light rolling motions upwards along the face.
- Start from the neck and move towards the forehead.
- Store in the fridge for an extra cooling effect.
- Use daily for 5 minutes.

Best For:

- Morning puffiness, dark circles, and skin relaxation.

Precautions:

- Be gentle around the eyes.
- Avoid rolling on active acne.

4. Facial Cupping – Skin Rejuvenation & Wrinkle Reduction

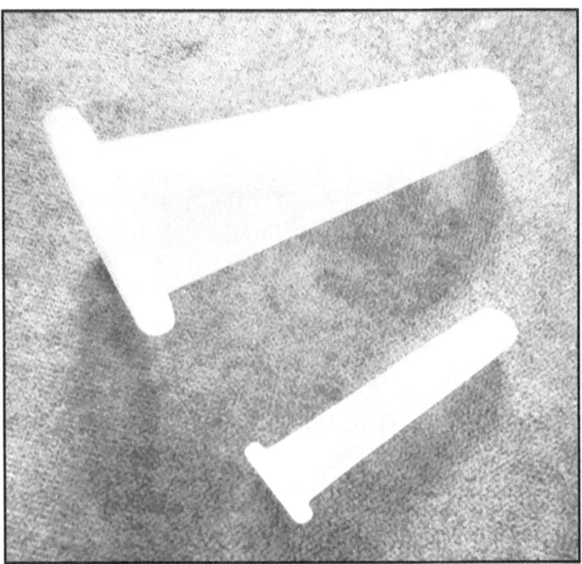

What It Is:

- Small silicone used to create gentle suction on the skin.
- Inspired by Chinese medicine, it boosts circulation and collagen production.

Benefits:

- Increases blood flow, making skin plumper and firmer
- Reduces fine lines and wrinkles
- Relieves muscle tension and detoxifies skin

How to Use It:

- Apply a facial oil for smooth movement.
- Squeeze the cup and place it on the skin, then gently glide in upward motions.
- Use smaller cups for delicate areas like under the eyes.
- Do this for 3–5 minutes a few times per week.

Best For:

- Fine lines, sagging skin, facial muscle relaxation.

Precautions:

- Avoid keeping cups in one spot for too long (can cause bruising).
- Don't use on broken or sensitive skin.

5. Face Taping – Instant Lift & Wrinkle Prevention

What It Is:

- A technique using adhesive tapes to lift and train facial muscles overnight.

Benefits:

- Smooths wrinkles overnight
- Prevents deep expression lines from forming
- Trains facial muscles to stay lifted

How to Use It:

- Clean and dry your face.
- Apply face tape along areas prone to wrinkles (forehead, nasolabial folds, jawline).
- Leave on overnight or for a few hours.

Best For:

- Forehead wrinkles, laugh lines, and sagging cheeks.

Precautions:

- Avoid cheap adhesives that can irritate the skin.
- Don't stretch the skin too hard while taping.

6. LED Light Therapy Mask – Advanced Anti-Aging

What It Is:

- A mask with LED lights that emit different wavelengths for skin repair and collagen production.

Benefits:

- Red light stimulates collagen and reduces wrinkles
- Blue light fights acne and calms inflammation
- Green light reduces pigmentation and brightens skin

How to Use It:

- Clean your face and apply a hydrating serum.
- Wear the LED mask for 10–15 minutes.
- Use 3–4 times per week for visible results.

Best For:

- Fine lines, sagging skin, acne, and pigmentation.

Precautions:

- Use protective eyewear to prevent eye strain.
- Avoid overuse to prevent skin sensitivity.

Final Comparison: Best Home Facial Tools for Anti-Aging

Tool	Best For	How Often	Key Benefit
Gua Sha	Sculpting, lifting, lymph drainage	Daily	Defines jawline & cheekbones
Dermaroller	Wrinkles, collagen boost	1-2x per week	Stimulates collagen & product absorption
Jade Roller	De-puffing, relaxation	Daily	Soothes & reduces inflammation
Facial Cupping	Blood circulation, lifting	2-3x per week	Reduces wrinkles & firms skin
Face Taping	Wrinkle prevention	Overnight	Trains muscles to prevent sagging
LED Mask	Anti-aging, pigmentation	3-4x per week	Reduces wrinkles & brightens skin

Using a combination of these tools alongside face yoga and massages will enhance your anti-aging routine naturally!

WHY BEAUTY SLEEP?

The Beauty of Sleep—How Rest Transforms Your Appearance

The Science Behind Beauty Sleep

We often hear the phrase "beauty sleep," but the connection between sleep and physical appearance goes far beyond just an old saying. Science has proven that sleep is essential for maintaining youthful, radiant skin, bright eyes, and a refreshed, vibrant look. From repairing damaged cells to reducing inflammation and enhancing collagen production, sleep plays a critical role in how we look and feel.

Inadequate sleep can lead to dull skin, dark circles, fine lines, and even premature aging. On the other hand, a good night's rest can make you appear healthier, more attractive, and even more symmetrical. Let's explore the powerful link between sleep and beauty.

How Sleep Affects Skin Health

1. Cellular Repair and Regeneration

During sleep, the body goes into repair mode. Skin cells regenerate, damaged tissues are repaired, and new cells are formed. This process is most active during the deepest stages of sleep, particularly between 10 p.m. and 2 a.m., when the body produces growth hormones responsible for cell regeneration.

Lack of sleep disrupts this cycle, leading to slower skin renewal and a build-up of dead skin cells, making the complexion look dull and tired. Over time, this can contribute to premature aging, uneven skin tone, and loss of elasticity.

2. Collagen Production and Wrinkle Prevention

Collagen is the protein that keeps skin plump, firm, and youthful. The body produces the most collagen while we sleep, helping to repair sun damage, scars, and fine lines. Without enough rest, the body releases cortisol, the stress hormone that breaks down collagen and elastin, leading to sagging skin and wrinkles.

When you consistently get 7-9 hours of quality sleep, your skin remains hydrated, resilient, and elastic, reducing the appearance of fine lines and signs of aging.

3. Reduced Puffiness and Dark Circles

A restless night often results in puffy eyes and dark circles, making you look exhausted. This happens because poor sleep leads to fluid retention, causing swelling around the eyes. In addition, sleep deprivation causes blood vessels to dilate, resulting in the appearance of dark under-eye circles.

Elevating your head slightly while sleeping and staying hydrated can help minimize puffiness, while ensuring you get enough rest will naturally prevent dark circles.

4. Balanced Hydration and Detoxification

While we sleep, our body balances hydration levels by flushing out excess toxins and delivering nutrients to the skin. Lack of sleep can lead to dehydration, making the skin appear dry, flaky, and irritated. Dehydrated skin also highlights wrinkles and fine lines, giving a more aged appearance.

A well-rested body, on the other hand, maintains optimal moisture levels, resulting in a natural, dewy glow.

The Role of Sleep in Hair and Nail Health

1. Stronger, Shinier Hair

Hair growth is closely linked to sleep because the follicles receive nutrients, minerals, and vitamins while the body is at rest. During deep sleep, the scalp absorbs oxygen and nutrients, helping to strengthen hair strands and reduce breakage.

Sleep deprivation leads to increased stress hormones, which can disrupt the hair growth cycle and lead to hair thinning, dullness, and even premature graying.

2. Healthy Nails

Just like skin and hair, nails benefit from sleep-induced cell regeneration and protein synthesis. Well-rested individuals tend to have stronger, healthier nails, while those who lack sleep may notice brittle, weak nails that break easily.

The Psychological Effects of Sleep on Beauty

Beyond the physical benefits, sleep enhances mood, confidence, and overall attractiveness. Studies have shown that well-rested individuals are perceived as more attractive than sleep-deprived ones. Rest improves posture, facial expressions, and even the way we carry ourselves, all of which contribute to a more beautiful and radiant appearance.

Additionally, when you are well-rested, you are more likely to engage in healthy habits, such as maintaining a skincare routine, eating nutritious foods, and exercising—all of which contribute to beauty from the inside out.

Tips for Getting Quality Beauty Sleep

1. Stick to a Sleep Schedule – Aim for 7-9 hours of sleep each night and maintain a consistent bedtime routine.
2. Sleep on a Silk Pillowcase – Silk reduces friction on the skin and hair, preventing wrinkles and hair breakage.
3. Keep Your Bedroom Cool and Dark – A comfortable sleep environment enhances melatonin production, improving sleep quality.
4. Avoid Screens Before Bed – Blue light from screens disrupts melatonin levels, making it harder to fall asleep.
5. Hydrate and Moisturize – Drink plenty of water and apply a night cream to keep your skin hydrated while you sleep.
6. Sleep on Your Back – Sleeping face-down or on your side can cause sleep lines and wrinkles over time.
7. Manage Stress – Meditation, deep breathing, or journaling before bed can help you relax and improve sleep quality.

Conclusion

Sleep is nature's most powerful beauty treatment. It repairs, rejuvenates, and restores the skin, hair, and nails, ensuring you wake up looking and feeling your best. Prioritizing quality sleep is the simplest and most effective way to enhance your natural beauty and maintain a youthful, glowing appearance for years to come.

So the next time you're tempted to sacrifice sleep for work, socializing, or entertainment, remember: your beauty depends on it.

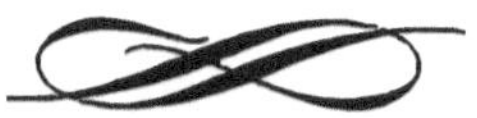

FINAL WORD: THE POWER OF FACE YOGA IN YOUR HANDS

As you reach the end of this journey into the world of face yoga, remember that true beauty is not just about looking youthful—it's about feeling confident, radiant, and in harmony with yourself. Face yoga is more than just a set of exercises; it's a daily ritual of self-care, a way to reconnect with your body, and a natural, empowering method to age gracefully.

Face yoga isn't just about physical transformation. It's about the energy you radiate when you take care of yourself. It's about self-love, self-discipline, and the joy of aging with grace. Every time you engage in these exercises, you're not just lifting your face; you're lifting your spirit, boosting your confidence, and embracing a more mindful way of living.

So, as you close this book, let this practice become a lifelong commitment—one that evolves with you, supports you, and reminds you daily that beauty is a reflection of your inner well-being. Trust in the process, stay consistent, and most importantly, enjoy the journey.

If you consistently activate and strengthen your facial muscles, they will support tight, lifted skin and a well-defined structure. The choice is yours—use it or lose it—but remember, a little effort today will keep your face youthful for years to come.

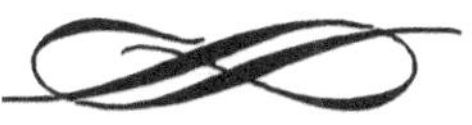

TESTIMONIAL

"I am a face yoga practitioner and teacher with Shubh Yoga Foundation, Rishikesh. I have been practicing face yoga since 2023 and I have got very good results. I lost my pregnancy fat on my cheeks and jawline. My skin is also looking younger still at this age. My face came in shape again. My face is my best testimonial for anyone who wants to do face yoga. Try it to believe it."

– Shachi Khemuka

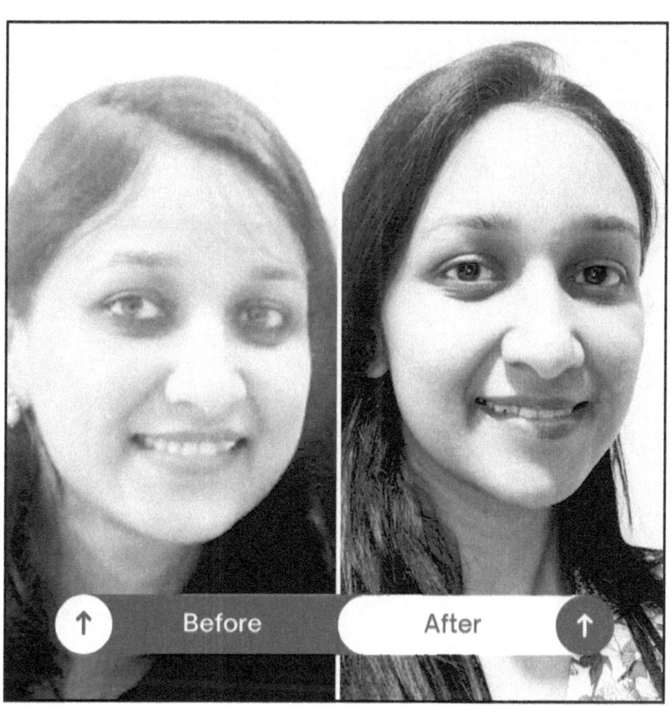